Essential Wound Management:
An introduction for undergraduates

Other titles available from Wounds UK include:

Honey: A modern wound management product
edited by Richard White, Rose Cooper and Peter Molan

Wound Healing: A systematic approach to advanced wound healing and management
edited by David Gray and Pam Cooper

A Pocket Guide to Clinical Decision-making in Wound Management
edited by David Gray and Sue Bale

Skin Care in Wound Management: Assessment, prevention and treatment
edited by Richard White

Wounds UK — The Directory, 2007 edited by Richard White and Clare Morris

The views expressed in this book are the views of the authors and are not the responsibility of Johnson & Johnson.

Essential Wound Management:
An introduction for undergraduates

David Gray, Pam Cooper and John Timmons

Wounds UK
—— Publishing ——

Johnson&Johnson
Wound Management

Wounds UK Publishing, Wounds UK Limited, Suite 3.1, 36 Upperkirkgate,
Aberdeen AB10 1BA   1005052 968

British Library Cataloguing-in-Publication Data
A catalogue record is available for this book

© Wounds UK Limited 2006
ISBN 0-9549193-2-7

Printed in the UK by Cromwell Press, Trowbridge, Wiltshire

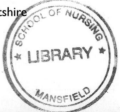

CONTENTS

LIST OF CONTRIBUTORS

Pam Cooper is a Clinical Nurse Specialist in Tissue Viability, Grampian NHS Acute Trust, Aberdeen.

David Gray is a Clinical Nurse Specialist in Tissue Viability, Grampian NHS Acute Trust, Aberdeen.

Andrew Kingsley is Tissue Viability Nurse Specialist, North Devon District Hospital, Barnstaple.

John Timmons is a Lecturer in Postgraduate Nursing, Glasgow Caledonian University.

Richard White is Senior Research Fellow, Department of Tissue Viability, Aberdeen Royal Infirmary, Aberdeen.

FOREWORD

Wounds have a huge impact on patients, their families and those involved in their treatment. Sound wound management and assessment will address not only wound-related problems, but also any concurrent illness with which the patient may present. The dramatic impact of wound healing and treatment on patients and their families, pushes practitioners and researchers to continue to expand their knowledge base.

This book, by combining the science with the more practical aspects of treating and caring for patients with wounds, introduces undergraduate healthcare practitioners to the field of wound management. Real patients with real wounds, who have been treated and managed by the authors are presented, bringing an individual, yet evidence-based approach to the topics covered.

The book itself is a journey from wound healing physiology through to utilising the most up-to-date wound assessment tools available.

The first chapter focuses on the physiology of wound healing and skin anatomy. Over the past two decades, much of the key research in wound healing has been rooted in our ability to examine this area with greater depth and understanding, developing therapies based on this new knowledge.

The second chapter examines the different types of wounds that we may encounter in practice, and provides excellent guidance on how to assess and manage such wounds.

The following chapter addresses the problem of the multifactorial nature of the patient with a chronic wound and discusses some of the intrinsic and extrinsic factors which can adversely affect the healing process, from age-related issues and diabetes to the role of nutrition. This chapter will help the reader to identify the potential problems in the wound healing process, and to set more realistic treatment goals based on the 'whole' patient, not just the wound.

Chapter 4 discusses the use of the Applied Wound Management system and how this can assist in wound management and treatment. By utilising the Wound Healing Continuum to identify tissue types, the reader is introduced to the Wound Infection Continuum, which assesses the bioburden of the wound in question. Finally, the Wound Exudate Continuum allows a more accurate and objective assessment of wound exudate levels. This is one of the most highly-regarded wound assessment tools available, which is invaluable when dealing with patients with different wound presentations.

With nursing curricula facing mounting pressure to include all possible patient issues, wound management in some areas may not receive the attention that it deserves. This book helps to fill that gap.

This publication maintains a patient focus throughout, providing a comprehensive review of wound management issues. It addresses the needs of undergraduate students and newly-qualified nurses alike, and is essential reading for all those involved in this fascinating and evolving area of practice.

John Timmons
Lecturer in Postgraduate/Post-registration Nursing
Glasgow Caledonian University
November, 2005

INTRODUCTION

Applied Wound Management is a method of wound assessment and documentation which seeks to facilitate clinical decision-making, communication between professionals, and clinical audit. This book is one of a number of tools which include, articles, journal supplements, clinical tools, clinical audit software, professional seminars and web-based resources which aim to support the practitioner in the use of Applied Wound Management. Applied Wound Management is a Wounds UK initiative, developed in partnership with Johnson and Johnson Advanced Wound Management.

David Gray
Clinical Director
Wounds UK
November, 2005

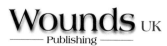

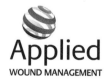

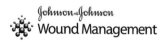

It is hoped that this book will reach into your practice and help you to reflect on how you currently manage patients with wounds, and assist you in improving and developing these skills.

To achieve this aim, the authors have developed reflective, self-assessment exercises at the end of each chapter to help you examine the themes and, by so doing, keep a record of wound management practice.

As a reflective document, these self-assessment exercises will be a useful addition to your portfolio, which may be used to satisfy the Nursing and Midwifery Council (NMC) guidelines. More importantly, this book, with such exercises, should help to provide you with an 'aide memoire' to guide your practice today and in the future.

John Timmons
Lecturer in Postgraduate/Post-registration Nursing
Glasgow Caledonian University
November, 2005

CHAPTER 1

WOUND HEALING PHYSIOLOGY

John Timmons

Introduction

Wound healing is an exciting and continually developing field, with new technologies and research playing a large part in improving the quality of patient care. The role of the nurse in wound care is all encompassing, stretching from the initial assessment of the wound and the patient, to making the correct decisions about treatment and beyond. Regular evaluation, and the setting of goals is essential to monitor the progress of the patient and the wound. However, to do this, a baseline knowledge of the functions and anatomy of the skin and wound healing physiology is required.

Functions of the skin

The skin, often referred to as the largest body organ, has six main functions:

❖ **Protection:** the skin serves as the main protective barrier, preventing damage to internal tissues from physical trauma, ultraviolet (UV) light, temperature changes, toxins and bacteria (Butcher and White, 2005). As well as preventing harmful substances from entering the body, it also controls the loss of vital substances (Graham-Brown and Burns, 1998).

❖ **Sensation:** the nerve endings present in the skin allow the body to detect pain, and changes in temperature, touch and pressure.

❖ **Thermoregulation:** the skin allows the body to respond to changes in temperature by constricting or dilating the blood vessels within it. The sweat glands produce sweat which stays on the skin allowing the body to cool down. When the body is cold, the hair erector pili contract, raising the hair and trapping warm air next to the skin.

❖ **Excretory function:** the skin excretes waste products in sweat which contains water, urea and albumin. Sebum is an oily substance which is excreted by the sebaceous glands, helping to lubricate and protect the skin.

❖ **Metabolism:** the skin produces vitamin D, which is required for calcium absorption when UV light is present.

❖ **Non-verbal communication:** the skin can convey changes in mood through colour changes such as blushing. The skin also gives clues as to our physical well-being (Flanagan and Fletcher, 2003).

The skin needs to remain intact to allow the body to perform these vital functions. When the skin is breached, it is important to close the defect as quickly as possible, thereby preventing infection from occurring and allowing normal skin function to return.

Anatomy and physiology of the skin

The skin consists of two main layers: the outermost region is the epidermis and the underlying region, the dermis. Beneath the dermis is the hypodermis.

Epidermis

The epidermis (*Figure 1.1*) consists mostly of tissue called stratified epithelium. Stratified epithelium consists of one or more layers of cells. Epithelium always has one free surface, which means that no other cells adhere to it. The opposite surface of the epithelium is a basement membrane. This is a non-cellular layer, rich in proteins and polysaccharides, that lies between the epithelium and the underlying connective tissue. The cells arise in the epidermis, but are pushed towards its free surface as rapid and ongoing cell division produces new cells beneath them.

Most cells of the epidermis are called keratinocytes. Each is a tiny factory for manufacturing keratin, a tough, water-insoluble protein. These cells start to produce keratin when they reach the mid-epidermal regions. By the time they reach the skin's free surface, they are dead and flattened.

The epidermis is divided into five layers: the stratum corneum (horny layer), stratum lucidum (clear layer), stratum granulosum (granular layer), stratum spinosum (prickle-cell layer), and stratum basale (basal layer). Sometimes the stratum spinosum and stratum basale are collectively known as the stratum germinativum.

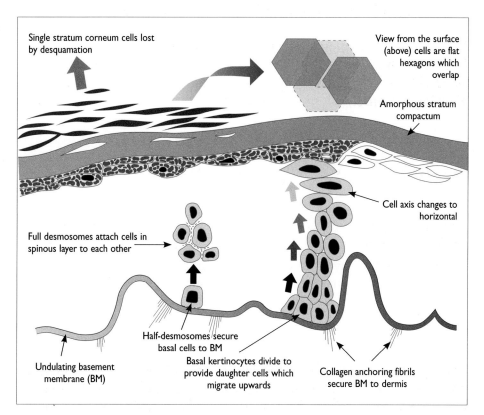

Figure 1.1: A diagrammatic view of the skin, illustrating key features of epidermal biology (Butcher and White, 2005)

Stratum corneum

This is the tough, waterproof, uppermost layer of the epidermis. The stratum corneum consists of dead cells which are fibrous in nature and contain keratin. The dead cells assist in the protective role of the skin by resisting certain chemicals and changes in pH and temperature. Millions of the cells are worn off daily, but cell divisions push up replacements continually. This contributes to the skin's ability to repair itself following trauma. Keratin is also capable of absorbing water which may lead to skin maceration from prolonged exposure to an excessively moist environment, eg. wound exudate, urine.

Stratum lucidum

This is a transparent layer of cells that are not always present, especially in areas of the body where the skin is thinner. This layer is thought to provide extra protection as it is present in areas exposed to wear and tear, such as the palms of the hand and soles of the feet.

Stratum granulosum

The stratum granulosum is the layer in which the keratinocytes lose their nuclei and begin to flatten and die, and where keratinisation starts to take place.

Stratum spinosum

Above the basal layer is the stratum spinosum. This layer of the epidermis contains living cells which contain spiny processes known as desmosomes. These assist in maintaining the integrity of the epidermis.

Stratum basale

This is the lowest layer of the epidermis, and is also known as the basement membrane. The stratum basale is one cell thick and forms a definite border between the dermis and the epidermis.

The basal cells which make up the stratum basale constantly divide, allowing the continuous regeneration of the skin. The daughter cells are slowly driven, by the active cell division, into the other layers of the epidermis where they undergo various development stages.

The stratum basale also controls the transfer of key proteins and oxygen between the dermis and epidermis, as the epidermis does not have a blood supply of its own. The stratum basale also supports the epidermis by fibrils which reach into the dermis.

Also scattered within this layer are specialised cells called melanocytes which make melanin, the brown substance that accumulates during a sun tan. We all have similar numbers of melanocytes, but those of dark-skinned people are genetically programmed to make far more melanin than those with fair skin.

Dermis

The primary function of the dermis is to provide support and nutrients to the epidermis. The two layers identified within the dermis are the papillary layer and the reticular layer.

The papillary layer, or stratum papillare, is the upper layer of the dermis, which is clearly demarcated from the epidermis by an undulated border. This wave-like structure increases the contact area with the epidermis, and ensures that the blood vessels of the dermis provide the stratum basale of the epidermis with optimal nourishment. The papillary layer consists of loose connective tissue, capillaries, elastic fibres, reticular fibres and collagen.

The thicker, reticular layer, or stratum reticulare, contains denser connective tissue, larger blood vessels, elastic fibres, and bundles of collagen arranged in layers.

The main constituent of the dermis is the proteinous connective tissue made up of arc-shaped, elastic fibres and undulated, nearly inelastic, collagen fibres. These are responsible for the high elasticity and tensile strength of the dermis, and fend off damage from everyday stretching and other mechanical insults.

Glycosaminoglycans (also known as mucopolysaccharides) bind with the proteinous connective tissue to form proteoglycans. These form a gel-like mass that can absorb and expel water like a sponge.

Other constituents of the dermis are various types of cells such as fibroblasts, mast cells and other tissue cells, as well as a multitude of blood and lymph vessels, nerve endings, hot and cold receptors, and tactile sensory organs.

Hypodermis

The hypodermis (also known as the superficial fascia), is a tissue that anchors the skin while allowing some freedom of movement. It provides support for the dermis and is made up of largely adipose tissue, connective tissue, and blood vessels. Fat stored in the hypodermis helps to protect internal structures and also provides insulation against cold.

Wound healing physiology

Wound healing physiology can be complex. The wound healing process can be affected by a number of external and internal influences. Therefore, when treating a patient with a wound, it is essential that a thorough patient history is taken and underlying conditions that could influence healing are diagnosed.

The main aim of the wound healing process is to restore the damaged area to normal strength and function (or as normal as possible). However, for some patients with wounds, particularly in palliative care settings, wound healing will not be the ultimate aim but, rather, improving their quality of life (Leaper and Harding, 1998).

Wounds are often divided into acute or chronic, and heal by primary or secondary intention.

Acute wounds are those which result from surgery or trauma, and usually have a relatively short, uneventful healing time. Burns, due to the area of tissue damage, will often behave more like chronic wounds.

Chronic wounds are wounds such as leg ulcers, pressure ulcers, diabetic foot ulcers, and malignant wounds. Chronic wounds tend to have prolonged healing times, are prone to episodes of infection, and may have increased levels of exudate due to prolonged inflammation.

Primary intention healing refers to a wound where the wound edges have been brought together by sutures, clips, staples or glue. There is often minimal tissue loss and the healing process is relatively short (*Chapter 2, p. 31*).

In secondary intention healing, there is an open wound, occasionally a cavity, which heals from the base of the wound and, in the latter stages, by contraction of the wound edges (*Chapter 2, pp. 31–32*).

When studying wound healing, it is important to remember that most descriptive models refer to the healing of acute wounds and the data is often extrapolated to include chronic wounds. Chronic wounds do not follow the normal sequence of events, hence their chronicity, so delays and interruptions to the healing process will be encountered. Healing is a dynamic process where the descriptive stages overlap and do not occur in isolation of each other.

The wound healing process can be divided into four main phases which do not occur in isolation: haemostasis, inflammation, proliferation and maturation (*Figure 1.2*). This means that it is difficult to place a definite time scale on the sequence of events (*Table 1.1*). It is also important to remember that in chronic wounds there will be large variations in the wound healing process, depending on the patient and the presentation of the wound.

Table 1.1: Wound healing times	
Stage of healing	Time scale
Haemostasis	Within approximately ten minutes
Inflammation	Approximately three days
Proliferation	Approximately twenty-eight days
Maturation	Up to a year or more

Haemostasis

Haemostasis, or the arrest of bleeding, describes the normal physiological response of the body following wounding. The volume of blood lost depends on the severity of the injury and the blood vessels involved. The cut surfaces of the blood vessels expose connective tissue which attracts platelets to the site of the injury. Platelets enter the area and, on coming into contact with collagen in the walls of the damaged blood vessels, stick together. This aggregation activates the platelets to release a number of agents (including platelet-derived growth factor [PDGF]) that trigger the clotting cascade (Silver, 1994). This results in initial vasoconstriction that reduces blood flow through the damaged vessels. As a result, the area surrounding the wound may appear pale.

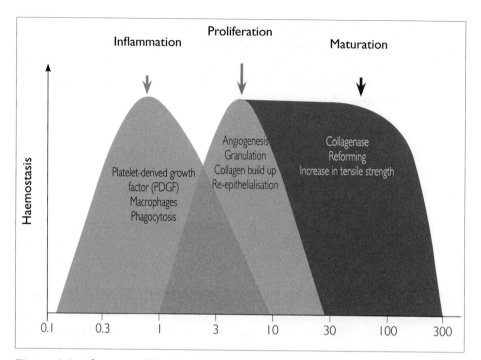

Figure 1.2: The wound healing process. This graph represents approximate timescales and illustrates the overlap that occurs during the healing process

Platelet aggregation and the release of bradykinin and histamine result in a build up of pressure within the capillary, causing the vessel to dilate. This can be viewed as erythema on the surface of the skin (Shields and O'Kane, 1994). The increase in blood flow helps to flush debris and bacteria from the wound, and the vessel dilation promotes the movement of fluid into the tissues. This response is observed at the wound site as redness, heat, and swelling. In most cases, approximately five to ten minutes after injury, the vessels are sealed and haemostasis is achieved.

Inflammation

It is important to realise that inflammation is a 'normal' vascular and cellular response to any kind of injury, not only a wound. Healing will not progress if the inflammatory response does not occur. The inflammatory phase of wound healing lasts approximately three to five days in acute wounds, but in chronic wounds can be protracted. The inflammatory phase begins as soon as the injury is sustained.

The release of PDGF and proteases assists in attracting chemical agents and cells to the area. This phase of wound healing is recognised by visible erythema, oedema, and increased heat which is a result of the increased blood flow to the area and the vessel wall permeability (Hart, 2002).

Inflammation is characterised by:

- redness (rubor)
- swelling (tumor)
- heat (calor)
- pain (dolor).

The rise in extracellular fluid as it passes through the vessel walls (extravasation) gives rise to oedema (swelling). The increase in blood flow brings with it a rise in local temperature (heat), and the increase in pressure from the volume of extracellular fluid leads to pain.

The extra blood flow resulting from vasodilation leads to extra white cells (neutrophils) at the site, which cleanse the wound area of bacteria and devitalised tissue. Monocytes are also attracted to the area by PDGF. Monocytes transform into macrophages which continue with the cleansing activity and are essential if healing is to progress (Leibovich and Ross, 1975). Macrophages secrete the proteases collagenase and elastase. These enzymes break down damaged tissue that is not required. Inflammatory exudate in a healthy wound contains many vital ingredients to assist the healing process. Two agents that are important for wound bed preparation (Falanga, 2002) include the proteases and neutrophils identified above. Although the presence of exudate is vital for cell activity, it can also damage intact skin, so exudate needs to be managed to prevent further breakdown in the wounded area.

Proteins of the complement system (so called because it complements the action of antibodies in the blood) are activated and stimulate the release of histamine, and also assist in the attack and destruction of microbes (Silver, 1994).

The proliferative phase

Vascular endothelial growth factor (VEGF) released by the macrophages stimulates the formation of new blood vessels (angiogenesis). The newly-formed blood vessels deliver oxygen and nutrients to the healing tissues.

Fibroblasts will start to divide and produce collagen which builds elasticity and strength in the wound. Together with glycosaminoglycans and proteoglycans they form a ground substance or extracellular matrix (ECM). The ECM supports the new and developing blood vessels and fills the intracellular spaces with collagen fibres. The deposition of the extracellular matrix, together with angiogenesis, comprises the granulation tissue.

In acute wounds, granulation tissue forms within three to five days of injury. This stage overlaps with the inflammatory phase of healing, which can be noted in wounds containing both sloughy and granulating tissue.

Healthy granulation tissue is moist and appears bright red in colour (*Figure 1.3*). Unhealthy granulation tissue may be dark in colour and may bleed easily, indicating possible infection and poor vascular supply to the tissue.

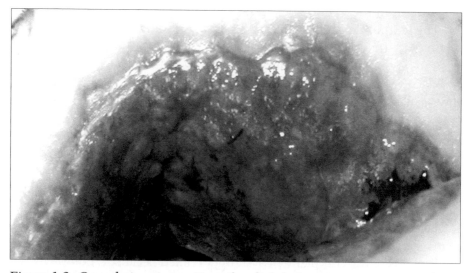

Figure 1.3: Granulation tissue. Note the slightly bumpy appearance and bright red colouration consistent with the laying down of new collagen and an increase in the vascularity of the tissue

Some fibroblasts change into specialist cells known as myofibroblasts, which begin to contract around the wound edges pulling them closer together. This process, known as contraction, is minimal in wounds which heal by primary intention but, due to the volume of tissue loss, is significant in wounds which heal by secondary intention. Once this has begun, re-epithelialisation will start to take place. New epithelial cells will begin to migrate from the edges of the wound and also from within hair follicles, sebaceous glands and sweat glands. The cells are white/pink in appearance and the layer is one cell thick once complete. The cells stop migrating once they have met other epithelial cells on the wound, by a process known as 'contact inhibition' (Garrett, 1998).

The new cells require the surface of the wound to be moist to allow this to occur. If the wound surface is allowed to dry out, the new cells must burrow underneath the dry tissue, which takes longer and there is a greater risk of infection.

Epithelialisation is influenced by the production of a number of growth factors (*Figure 1.4*). Macrophages produce keratinocyte growth factor (KGF) and this stimulates keratinocyte proliferation and migration through the extracellular matrix. The rate of epithelialisation is under the influence of epidermal growth factor (EGF) and transforming growth factor-β (TGF-β) (Tredget *et al*, 2005).

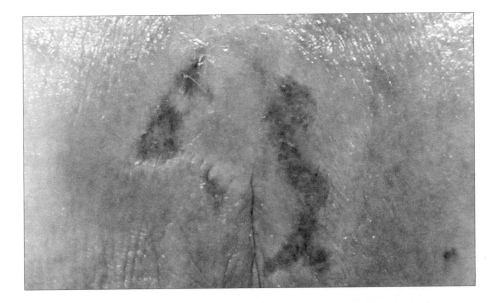

Figure 1.4: Epithelial tissue. During epithelialisation keratinocytes cover the wound from the edges and in islands from which they grow, due to their production in hair follicles, sweat glands and sebaceous glands

Maturation

The maturation phase of wound healing may take up to eighteen months to complete (Silver, 1994). This phase is sometimes known as the remodelling phase of healing and, during this time, the wound is strengthened and the scar will change colour significantly.

Collagen bundles within the wound, which were once laid down in an irregular fashion, mature to form a stronger, more organised layer. In addition, the vascular network will decrease which may leave the scar looking less red and, in many cases, the scar appears 'silver' or white in colour. The scar itself is relatively avascular and will not support hair follicles, sweat glands or sebaceous glands.

For many, the process of healing is straightforward, however, for a number of patients with chronic wounds, healing can be prolonged by factors which may relate to the type of wound, or, to the patient's general well-being. By understanding the physiology of normal wound healing and its relevant stages, we are better placed to intervene and provide management and treatment solutions when problems occur.

References

Butcher M, White R (2005) The structure and functions of the skin. In: White R, ed. *Skin Care in Wound Management: Assessment, prevention and treatment*. Wounds UK, Aberdeen

Falanga V (2002) Wound bed preparation and the role of enzymes; a case for multiple actions of therapeutic agents. *Wounds* **14**(2): 47–57

Flanagan M, Fletcher J (2003) Tissue Viability: Managing chronic wounds. In: Booker C, Nicol M, eds. *Nursing Adults: The practice of caring*. Mosby, St Louis

Garrett B (1998) Re-epithelialisation. *J Wound Care* **7**(7): 358–9

Graham-Brown R, Burns T (1998) *Lecture Notes on Dermatology*. 7th edn. Blackwell Science, Oxford

Hart (2002) Inflammation 1: its role in the healing of acute wounds. *J Wound Care* **11**(6): 205–8

Leaper DJ, Harding KG (1998) *Wounds, Biology and Management*. Oxford University Press, Oxford

Leibovich SJ, Ross R (1975) The role of the macrophage in wound repair: a study with hydrocortisone and anti-macrophage serum. *Am J Pathology* **78**(1): 71–100

Shields D, O'Kane S (1994) Laser photobiomodulation of wound healing. In: Baxter ED, ed. *Therapeutic Lasers*. Churchill Livingstone, Edinburgh

Silver JA (1994) The physiology of wound healing. *J Wound Care* **3**(2): 106–9

Tredget EB, Demare J, Chandran G (2005) Transforming growth factor-beta and its effect on re-epithelialisation. *Wound Rep Regen* **13**(1): 61–7

Self-assessment exercises

The patients you see in practice may have wounds at various stages of the healing process:

❖   Inflammation
❖   Proliferation
❖   Maturation

Consider what is going on in the wounds at each stage and reflect on how this affects your treatment of the wound.

How does your product selection differ with each change in the phase of healing?

During the inflammatory phase, we consider using products which may assist in debridement of sloughy tissue, absorption of exudate and reduction in the risk of infection.

Which products may perform these functions?

In the proliferative phase we may use products which will offer some physical protection to the newly-growing granulation tissue and not adhere to the wound bed. Bacterial barriers are also important at this stage.

Which products would be ideal to protect the wound at this stage?

In the maturative phase most wounds will be exposed, however, there is a loss of tensile strength area which may predispose the patient to further injury. Hypertrophic scarring in some patients may also occur and there are products available which can reduce the size and colour of such scars.

Which products might you use?

CHAPTER 2

A REVIEW OF DIFFERENT WOUND TYPES AND THEIR PRINCIPLES OF MANAGEMENT

Pam Cooper

Introduction

Wounds can be categorised into many different groups and sub-groups according to their wide and varied pathologies. However, it is possible to categorise most wounds healing by secondary intention into the following six categories; pressure ulcers, leg ulcers, diabetic foot ulcers, trauma wounds, surgical wounds and complex wounds. Before embarking on any plan of care, it is vital that the practitioner understands the cause of the wound and considers into which of the above categories the wound fits. An understanding of the basic principles of each type of wound is also essential to ensure well-informed clinical decision-making.

The three Wound Continuums, Healing, Infection and Exudate (*Chapter 4, p. 76*) provide a framework for assessing a wound in a systematic manner. However, it is essential that when assessing a wound, the practitioner understands the underlying pathology of the wound to accurately inform clinical decision-making. Such an understanding, combined with key management principles for the wound, be it a pressure, leg, or diabetic foot ulcer, can greatly enhance the level of care provided. For example, in the case of a pressure ulcer, removing the cause, eg. an inappropriate seat cushion, can prevent further damage and facilitate healing.

This chapter presents a brief overview of common wound types and the key principles for their management.

Pressure ulcers

Pressure ulcers (pressure sores, decubitus ulcers, bedsores) are areas of tissue death, usually located over a bony prominence, which have been caused by external forces of pressure, shear and friction (Allman, 1997). These may be further exacerbated by complications arising from the individual's physical condition, such as altered nutrition, excess moisture, etc (Maklebust, 1987).

* **Pressure** is the major causative factor in the development of pressure ulcers. The damage occurs when the body's soft tissue is compressed between a bony prominence and a hard surface, which occludes the blood supply, leading to tissue ischaemia and death.

* **Shear** usually occurs when the individual slides down the bed, the skeleton and close tissue move but the skin on the buttocks remains in the same place. This usually leads to the development of more extensive tissue damage.

* **Friction** occurs when two surfaces move or rub across one another, leading to superficial skin loss.

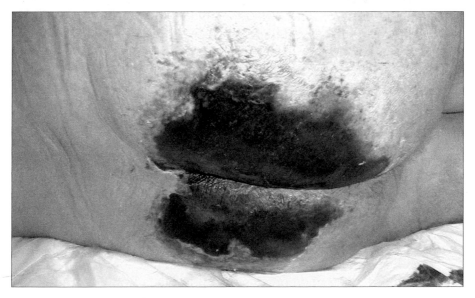

Figure 2.1: Pressure ulcer to sacrum

The care of those individuals who are either at risk of pressure ulcer development, or with existing pressure ulcers, should be based on prevention of pressure ulcers or the management/treatment of existing pressure ulcer damage. This approach should be holistic, focusing on the individual as a whole.

Physical assessment

❖ **General health:** Bliss (1990) suggests that acutely ill individuals are particularly vulnerable to the development of pressure ulcers, although the reasons for this are uncertain. If there has been a change in the individual's condition through illness, this should be considered when assessment of risk is carried out.

❖ **Age:** the majority of pressure ulcers recorded are found in the elderly, those over sixty-five years of age. This may be due to changes in their physical condition and skin. The skin loses its natural elasticity and becomes thinner, making it more susceptible to damage (*Chapter 3, pp. 51–52*).

❖ **Reduced mobility:** this reduces the individual's ability to alter position and to relieve pressure, be it in bed or while sitting up, thus making them more susceptible to the effects of sustained pressure.

❖ **Nutritional status:** this impairs the elasticity of the skin, reducing its ability to sustain the effects of pressure, shear and friction without leading to tissue breakdown (*Chapter 3, pp. 56–57*).

❖ **Incontinence:** it is now generally recognised that incontinence has a significant impact on the development of pressure ulcers, due to the combined effects of moisture, friction and pressure. Jordan *et al* (1977) found that 15.5% of patients with pressure ulcers were incontinent of urine, and 39.7% were incontinent of faeces.

Skin has a mean pH of 5.5 which is slightly acidic. Both urine and faeces are alkaline in nature, therefore, if the individual is incontinent, there is an immediate chemical reaction. Ammonia is produced when microorganisms rupture urea from the urine. Although urinary ammonia alone is not a primary irritant, urine and faeces together increase the pH at the peri-anal area, prompting the faecal irritant effect (Leyden _et al_, 1977; Berg, 1986). This is responsible for the dermatitis excoriation seen in individuals with incontinence (Fiers, 1996). The increase in moisture from episodes of incontinence, combined with bacterial and enzymatic activity, can cause the breakdown of vulnerable skin, due to an increased friction co-efficient, particularly in the very young or elderly.

❖ **Poor blood supply:** patients with evidence of poor blood supply, particularly to the peripheries such as the foot, have an increased risk of pressure damage. The effect of sustained low pressure on an already compromised limb can lead to the development of extensive tissue damage over a very short period of time. Particular attention should be paid when caring for these patients.

Risk assessment

To consider preventing pressure ulcers we must first determine an individual's risk of pressure ulcer development. All risk assessment tools are based on factors known to predispose an individual to pressure ulcer development, such as sustained pressure, reduced mobility, incontinence, poor nutrition, age, mental alertness and poor physical condition. There are a number of risk assessment tools available to select from; Norton (1962), Gosnell (1973), Towey and Erland (1988), Waterlow (1984) and Braden (1985). All of which have a research-based rationale dependent on their patient population. However, it should be remembered that they are to be used as an 'aide memoir' alongside clinical judgement and experience. Any intervention adopted following risk assessment should be clearly recorded in the individual's health records.

Skin inspection

It is essential that skin inspections are carried out to determine what is normal reactive hyperaemia, and what is abnormal non-blanching hyperaemia.

❖ **Reactive hyperaemia** – the characteristic bright flush of the skin associated with the release of pressure, a direct response to incoming blood.

❖ **Non-blanching hyperaemia** – there is no skin colour change when light finger pressure is applied, indicating an alteration to the blood supply and an initial sign of pressure damage.

Table 2.1 shows how to assess if the changes to the skin are a result of pressure damage.

Table 2.1: Skin assessment
Further examination of erythema should include the following:
• Apply light finger pressure to the area for ten seconds
• Release the pressure. If the area is white and then returns to its original colour, the area probably has an adequate blood supply. Observation should continue and preventative strategies should be employed
• If, on release of pressure, the area remains the same colour as before pressure was applied, it is an indication of the beginning of pressure ulcer development and preventative strategies should be employed
• If there is an alteration in skin colour (red, purple or black), or increased heat or swelling, it may imply underlying tissue breakdown. Frequency of assessment should be increased
• With dark skin pigmentation, pressure ulcer development will be indicated by areas where there is localised heat, or where there is damage, coolness, purple/black discoloration, localised oedema and induration

Pressure ulcer grading

If following skin inspection, pressure damage is observed, this should be recorded using an appropriate grading system. The grading of the pressure ulcer determines the degree of tissue damage, assisting the clinician to determine the type and level of clinical intervention required. Although this is not without a thorough wound assessment as well. There are a number of grading tools available which assess the degree of tissue involvement, namely:

- European Pressure Ulcer Advisory Panel (EPUAP, 2002) – A guide to pressure ulcer grading
- Stirling pressure sore severity scale (SPSSS, 1994)
- Torrance pressure sore grading scale (1983)
- Pressure ulcer scale for healing (PUSH, 2001).

Once the pressure ulcer has been graded, the individual or their carer is able to start the appropriate treatment and set up the correct interventions.

Table 2.2: Principles of management of pressure ulcers
• Prevention is better than treatment. If the individual is at risk of pressure ulcer development, ensure that appropriate preventative strategies have been adopted
• If a pressure ulcer has occurred, identify, remove, or treat the cause
• Treat the wound following the principles of the Wound Healing Continuum, based on accurate classification and wound assessment
• Ensure that the individual is cared for on an appropriate support surface while in bed and sitting up, according to the location of the pressure ulcer
• Ensure that the individual's underlying physical condition does not affect his/her ability to heal, ie. poor nutritional status

Positioning

Individuals at risk of, or with existing pressure ulcers, should have their position changed to reduce the effects of pressure. This should not be based on ritualistic practice, but on skin assessment and the individual's needs (Roycroft–Malone, 2000).

The use of turning regimes, such as the 30° tilt, has been effective at reducing tissue damage (Young, 2004) without the need to physically turn the individual. This is achieved not by moving or lifting the individual, but by using pillows to alter their position.

Individuals at risk of, or with pressure ulcers, should always be nursed on the appropriate support surfaces. Also, they should not be up for long periods, with evidence suggesting a maximum of one hour before returning to bed for a minimum of two hours (Defloor, 1999; Gebhardt and Bliss, 1994).

Equipment — mattresses and seating

Mattresses

Over recent years, the market has been filled with a wide variety of support surfaces designed to reduce the effects of pressure, shear and friction. These can be divided into two categories: static mattress systems and alternating/dynamic systems.

* **Static systems:** these are high quality cut foams, visco-elastic foams, or static air-filled systems. They reduce the effects of pressure by contouring to the individual's shape, redistributing the pressure across a much larger surface area. They do not require a power unit for operation.

* **Alternating/dynamic systems:** these provide alternating or low air-loss, which reduces the pressure at the individual's bony prominences. The alternating systems work by alternating their cells over a specific period of time. The vast majority of these beds will self-adjust to the individual's weight, although they have a minimum and maximum weight within which they operate. They are power activated.

Seating

* **Chairs:** individuals are at a greater risk of developing a pressure ulcer while sitting up, as 75% of their body weight is being transferred through the relatively small surface area of the buttocks (Günnewicht and Dunford, 2004). An individual at risk of pressure damage, who needs to be seated, should have an appropriate

cushion on their chair or wheelchair to offer protection to the pressure areas. If sitting in a chair, the height should be considered, as if the chair is either too low or too high, an increased pressure is placed on both the sacrum and the heels.

❖ **Cushions**: the range of cushions has increased, leading to the development of cut foams, visco-elastic foams, gel inserts, static and alternating air systems. The individual should be fitted for the appropriate cushion, considering height, weight and postural alignment. Occupational therapists, if available, may be able to help.

The management of pressure ulcers is often complex and fraught, with attention being focused on treating the wound. However, when caring for an individual with a pressure ulcer, the key prevention and management principles should be considered.

Leg ulcers

Chronic leg ulcers are a major health problem within the UK, primarily affecting the elderly patient population. It has been suggested that 80% of these are being cared for within the community environment (Cornwall *et al*, 1986), increasing the demands on already stretched resources.

A chronic leg ulcer is defined as an open lesion between the knee and the ankle joint that remains unhealed for at least four weeks (Scottish Intercollegiate Guidelines Network [SIGN], 1998).

The assessment of the individual and the leg ulcer should be comprehensive. The individual's co-morbidity must be assessed as this may greatly influence the treatment's aims and objectives. The assessment should consider if the leg ulcer is arterial, venous, or mixed in aetiology, and should also exclude factors such as rheumatoid arthritis and systemic vasculitis, as well as diabetic lesions.

Leg ulcer assessment

Historically, the most common method of leg ulcer assessment has been the traditional Doppler assessment. However, the technique requires considerable skill and expertise, which can prove difficult for nurses to maintain as the test is rarely requested. This has led to the work being carried out using pulse oximetry and the development of the Lanarkshire oximetry index (LOI).

Doppler assessment

Measurement of ankle brachial pressure ratio (index) (ABPI) by hand-held Doppler is essential in the assessment of chronic leg ulcers (SIGN, 1998). This is based on the Doppler probe being held over the vein, the blood pressure cuff being inflated, and once the Doppler signal disappears this is your recorded value. The brachial systolic pressure recorded in the arm is used as the baseline recording, and then the posterior tibial and dorsalis pedis are recorded in the feet.

The ABPI is calculated for each leg by dividing the highest ankle systolic pressure of each leg by the higher of the two brachial pressures (Jones, 2000).

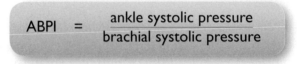

$$ABPI = \frac{\text{ankle systolic pressure}}{\text{brachial systolic pressure}}$$

* Pressures of 0.5–0.8 indicate evidence of significant arterial impairment (0.5 = 50% reduction in arterial blood flow).
* Pressures of 0.6–0.7 may have reduced compression if it has been assessed and applied by an experienced trained leg ulcer care expert (Royal College of Nursing [RCN], 1998).
* Pressures of 0.8 and above are suitable for compression (RCN, 1998). Caution should be taken with patients with diabetes and in patients with arteriosclerosis, as abnormally high readings might be caused by calcified arteries (Pudner, 1998).

Lanarkshire oximetry index (LOI)

The Lanarkshire oximetry index uses the method of pulse oximetry to measure the oxygen saturation of haemoglobin in blood or tissue, by detecting the amount of infrared light absorbed. However, like Doppler, it also depends on the presence of pulsatile blood flow in the arteries. This is carried out in a similar method to Doppler with the use of a blood pressure cuff, but instead of trying to find vessels, the probe is placed on one of the investigating limb's digits. The cuff is inflated initially to 60 mmHG, then inflated in 10 mmHG increments with ten seconds between each increment. When the pulse is lost, the pressure reading one below is recorded. A baseline recording is carried out on the arm and then the legs are investigated. The LOI is calculated as: LOI = toe pressure divided by finger pressure. Studies have suggested that LOI is at least as effective as Doppler (Bianchi, 2005), but it may have limitations in individuals with grossly dystrophic toe nails, extreme cyanosis, or in conditions where peripheral vascular constriction is evident.

Below are four of the most prevalent types of lower extremity wounds encountered in clinical practice.

Venous leg ulcers

Chronic venous insufficiency is due to impaired drainage in the venous system, with subsequent venous hypertension. Common sites for venous leg ulcers are above the medial malleoli and above the lateral malleoli.

Visual assessment of the skin and lower leg

On inspection, venous leg ulcers tend to be shallow in appearance without punched out wound margins located above the malleoli. Classic signs of venous leg ulceration are:

❖ **Varicose veins:** these are a clear indication of chronic venous hypertension in the lower limb, which is usually due to damage of the vessels there. About 3% of individuals with varicose veins go on to develop venous leg ulcers (Morison and Moffat, 1994).

❖ **Ankle flare:** chronic venous hypertension can cause distension of the tiny veins in the medial aspect of the foot. On inspection, it presents as purple blood vessel distoration, often referred to as ankle flare.

❖ **Lipodermatosclerosis:** the characteristic brown staining of the lower leg is suggestive of chronic venous disease. This occurs later on as progressive deposits of fibrous tissue in the deep dermis and fat result in the woody induration of the gaiter area of the shin.

❖ **Atrophie blanche:** this is often associated with irregular pigmentation, and presents as white areas of extremely thin skin dotted with tiny tortuous blood vessels.

❖ **Eczema:** this is commonly known as stasis dermatitis, and may appear in the gaiter area.

Visual inspection of the limb and a diagnostic assessment, ie. Doppler or LOI, should confirm if the limb is venous in nature. Once correct diagnosis is determined, treatment can be established.

Treatment

Patients with venous ulceration (ABPI >0.8) should have some form of elastic graduated compression applied with a simple non-adherent dressing to the wound. This may be a multi-layered bandage system (SIGN, 1998) or some form of compression hosiery (Best Practice Statement for Compression Hosiery, 2005). Therapeutic compression should provide a minimum of 30 mmHg–40 mmHg pressure at the ankle.

Arterial leg ulcers

Arterial ulcers are less common than those caused by venous disease, but arterial insufficiency, if present, complicates the healing of the wound. Arterial ulcers are caused by an insufficient arterial blood supply to the lower limb, resulting in tissue ischaemia and necrosis. Atherosclerosis is by far the commonest cause of venous insufficiency. Atherosclerosis reduces the blood flow to the lower limbs, and the degree of ischaemia and symptoms experienced depend not only on the site of occlusion, but also on the circulation above and below the occlusion site. At rest, an individual may be able to tolerate occlusion without experiencing any significant symptoms. However, during exercise, the increased demand for oxygen which cannot be met, can lead to intermittent claudication so that the person has to stop and rest because of the lack of blood supply to the muscles.

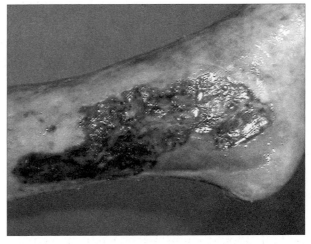

Figure 2.2: Arterial leg ulcer

The majority of patients with claudication have an ABPI between 0.8 and 0.4, while patients with rest pain have an ABPI of <0.4 (Sumner, 1989).

Identified risk factors for arterial disease include smoking or tobacco use, hyperlipidaemia, diabetes, hypertension, obesity, advanced age, trauma, sickle cell disease, and cardiovascular disease.

Visual assessment of the skin and lower leg

When visually inspecting a limb thought to have an arterial ulcer, the following should be considered:

❖ **The ulcer itself:** arterial ulcers are mainly found on the anterior shin, over toe joints, over malleoli and under the heel. They usually present as a large area of tissue loss, often circumferential with deep wound edges, and are often described as a 'dog taking a bite'. They are usually very painful and individuals find dressing changes difficult — pain control is paramount. The limb is often hairless.

❖ **Poor pallor:** when the patient is lying flat in their bed, the poor pallor of their foot is an indication of ischaemia.

❖ **Dusky red or cyanotic blue appearance of the skin:** this occurs in some cases, where impaired perfusion has resulted in blood stagnation within dilated arterioles (Foster and Edmons, 1987).

Treatment

If an arterial ulcer is diagnosed, the individual should be immediately referred to a vascular surgeon. This is to determine if any surgical intervention can be carried out to improve perfusion and the blood supply to the limb. If surgery is not an option, due to the individual or their physical condition, conservative management is recommended. Where the wound requires dressing, it is generally felt that moist wound healing can predispose the individual to infection and healing will be compromised. This is due to poor perfusion and, therefore, the area is usually kept dry and infection free.

Mixed venous/arterial ulcers

These ulcers will have the features of a venous ulcer in combination with signs of arterial impairment (RCN, 1998)

A full lower leg assessment should be performed and if the ABPI is reduced (for example, <0.8), the patient should be referred for a routine vascular referral (RCN, 1998). To treat the venous component of the disease, and promote wound healing without causing further ischaemia or injury, use of reduced compression at levels of 23 mmHg to 30 mmHg is indicated if the ABPI is 0.6–0.8. The patient should be carefully monitored in these circumstances, paying particular attention to the correct application of compression to ensure that tissue injury does not occur (Bonham, 2003).

When carrying out assessments on the lower limb, the clinician should also consider the following co-morbidities during diagnosis.

Rheumatoid arthritis and systemic vasculitis

Individuals diagnosed with rheumatoid arthritis and systemic vasculitis are prone to leg ulceration. This is due to the skin over the tibial area being poorly vascularised. Trauma, or a vasculitic episode, can lead to the sudden occurrence of a lesion, which can deteriorate rapidly and be slow to heal. It is, however, generally recognised, that the aetiology of ulcers in patients with rheumatoid arthritis is not always clear (Cawley, 1987).

Vasculitic ulcers usually present as small, painful, multiple ulcers, with no indication of chronic venous hypertension. They are usually associated with inflammatory connective disorders such as polyarteritis nodosa and systemic lupus erythematosus (Morison and Moffat, 1994). Diagnosis can be difficult and specialist referral is recommended.

Due to the complex nature of the underlying disease processes, the healing of these wounds depends on the disease treatment and can be slow.

Table 2.3: Principles of management of leg ulcers

- All individuals with a leg ulcer should be assessed in line with national clinical guidelines

- A Doppler and/or LOI assessment of the circulation should be carried out by a skilled practitioner, and individuals with abnormal readings referred to a specialist

- Compression therapy remains the treatment of choice for venous leg ulceration

- Arterial leg ulceration should be referred for further vascular assessment. This is required to establish the extent of the occlusion and the presence of small vessel disease. A specialist assessment will determine whether the patient is suitable for angioplasty or major vascular surgery

- In mixed ulceration, features of venous ulcers in combination with signs of arterial impairment require assessment by an experienced practitioner. The person conducting the assessment should be aware that ulcers may be arterial, diabetic, rheumatoid or malignant, and refer the patient for specialist medical assessment (RCN, 1998). Reduced compression therapy should only be carried out by a competent practitioner

- Due to the complex nature of diabetic lower leg ulceration, it is advisable to obtain specialist referral by the multidisciplinary team and ensure a specialist Doppler assessment and the involvement of the diabetologist

Diabetes and neuropathy

Atherosclerosis is common in people with diabetes. It occurs bilaterally, and affects the microvascular as well as larger vessels. Individuals with long-term diabetes commonly suffer from sensory, motor, and autonomic neuropathy, due to impaired nerve function from hyperglycaemia. The combination of poor perfusion, altered sensation, and motor/nerve-induced foot deformity from neuropathy, results in limited joint mobility and gait alteration, which causes abnormal stress and pressure on the foot and leads to callus development. This increased pressure results in ulceration which, far too often in patients with diabetes, can cause infection, gangrene, and limb loss. Wound infection is particularly troublesome because it can occur without the individual's awareness of the usual signs of pain, swelling, and erythema, resulting in an extensive infection before it is recognised (Cooper *et al*, 2004).

Diabetic wounds

Diabetes is a common health condition. About 1.4 million people in the UK are known to have diabetes — that's about three in every 100 people. Diabetic foot ulcer management is complex in nature with a high rate of amputation. In a two-year retrospective study in Gwent, they had an amputation prevalence rate of 7% for diabetic patients (De *et al*, 2000). This has a huge psychosocial impact on the patient, as well as cost implications. Krentz *et al* (1997) estimated an annual hospital cost of £400,000 in a prospective survey conducted.

Diabetic foot wounds present as a significant clinical management challenge and carry high complication risks. Individuals with diabetic ulceration may have deceptively high pressure readings and, as such, should be referred for specialist assessment. Their ulcers are usually found on the foot, and often on bony prominences such as the bunion area or under the metatarsal heads, and they tend to be sloughy or necrotic in appearance (Cullum and Roe, 1995).

Patients with diabetes may have neuropathic, arterial and/or venous components (Browse *et al*, 1988; Nelzen *et al*, 1993). Consequently, all patients with diabetes with leg ulcers require a multidisciplinary approach to care, ensuring that the appropriate specialist referrals are made. It is essential that a diabetologist is involved in this process. Patients with type 2 diabetes have a three- to five-fold increased risk of developing peripheral arterial disease, compared to people without diabetes (Shearman and Chulakadabba, 1999; Hurst and Lee, 2003). For those individuals with peripheral arterial disease and diabetes, the risk of myocardial infarction and stroke are raised, and the rate of amputation is increased by as much as seven times (Dormandy and Murray, 1991).

Painful diabetic neuropathy symptoms are often slight at first. Some mild cases may go unnoticed for a long time. Numbness, pain, or tingling in the feet or legs may, after several years, lead to weakness in the muscles of the feet. Occasionally, diabetic neuropathy can flare up suddenly and affect specific nerves, and the patient will develop double vision or drooping eyelids, or weakness and atrophy of the thigh muscles. The loss of sensation in the feet may increase the possibility for foot injuries to go unnoticed and develop into ulcers or lesions that become infected.

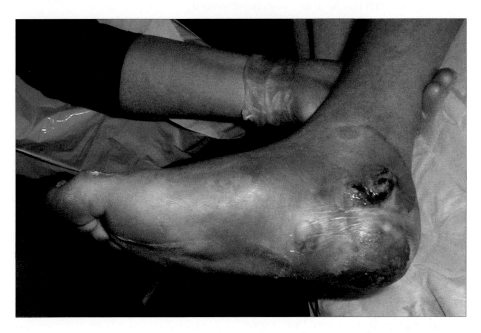

Figure 2.3: Diabetic foot ulcer, with cellulitis and osteomyelitis

Treatment

To ensure appropriate and effective treatment of this complex wound, the involvement of the whole multidisciplinary team is required. If the individual is experiencing pain, this should be addressed with an appropriate analgesic regime.

The wound should be assessed thoroughly, and any indication of infection should be eradicated with a topical antimicrobial and antibiotics (Benbow _et al_, 2004; Gray _et al_, 2003).

A full assessment should also determine the extent of the vascular/ nerve damage, and whether surgical intervention is required. The involvement of the podiatrist is essential to ensure correct shoeing and orthotic devices.

Table 2.4: Principles of management of diabetic wounds

- Diabetic foot wounds present a significant clinical management challenge and carry a high risk for those who suffer from them

- The two main features of foot ulceration are ischaemia and neuropathy, both of which predispose the individual to infection and lead to necrosis of the tissue

- Ensure the appropriate analgesia and antidepressants are prescribed for painful diabetic neuropathy (Benbow *et al*, 1999)

- Appropriate specialist referral should be made if the wound is infected

- Due to its complicated nature, a multidisciplinary approach to patient care is required when this problem manifests itself

---

Surgical wounds

There are many varied surgical techniques that can result in the development of a wound, such as:

- incisions or excisions
- investigative or corrective surgery
- open or keyhole surgery.

The following four types of wound healing are generally recognised (Thomas, 1990):

- primary closure, healing by first intention
- open granulation, healing by secondary intention
- delayed or secondary closure, sometimes called healing by third intention or tertiary intention
- grafting or flap formation.

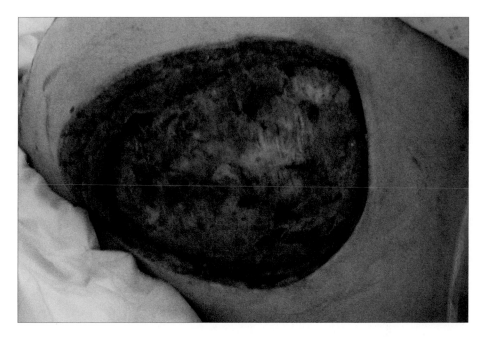

Figure 2.4: Surgical wound (abdominal cavity)

Healing by primary intention

Most clean surgical wounds are managed by primary closure. In this technique, the surgeon approximates the edges of the wound and individually sutures the different layers of tissue together. Primary closure is achieved by using either sutures, staples, Steri-Strips™ (3M™), tissue adhesives or a combination of all of these (Cooper *et al*, 2004). These wounds usually seal within twenty-four to forty-eight hours, and heal in eight to ten days when removal of sutures or staples takes place at the discretion of the surgeon. These wounds are usually covered in a low-adherent island dressing for the first twenty-four to forty-eight hours, and then are left exposed.

Healing by secondary intention

Secondary intention is often indicated in wounds that have sustained a degree of tissue loss as a result of surgery, or where an area has been excised and drained, due to abscess formation or pilonoidal sinus excision. Primary closure may be considered undesirable or impossible because of the extent of tissue loss, which makes it difficult to bring the edges of the wound together, or where pus may still be present, making the recurrence of infection high if primary closure were to be carried out. In these situations, the surgeon may favour leaving the wound open to heal by secondary intention. The duration of healing will vary in each individual case; wound healing is often affected by intrinsic and extrinsic factors that may result in complications (Baxter, 2003). As with all dressing choices, the primary function of a wound dressing is to promote healing by maintaining a moist wound environment. If healing by secondary intention, each dressing needs to be tailored to the size, depth, position and exudate level of the wound.

Healing by tertiary intention

Delayed primary closure is rather less commonly used. This occurs when the surgeon asserts that primary closure may be unsuccessful at the time of surgery, due to infection, poor blood supplies, or the need for excessive tension during closure. Patients will usually return for primary closure three to four days later. During this time, the dressing choice will be similar to that when left to heal by secondary intention.

Grafting or flap formation

A skin graft is an area of skin that is surgically removed from one part of the body and transplanted to another. The skin graft replaces tissue that has been destroyed, or creates new tissue where none exists. The major disadvantage of this technique is that another wound is created from the donor site. The most common types of skin grafts are partial-thickness or split skin grafts. These are removed from a suitable donor site, such as the thigh or buttock; donor sites usually heal rapidly within ten to fourteen days. Full-thickness skin grafts are used for more specialist surgery, where fat, hair, and sebaceous glands, are removed for transplanting.

Skin flaps usually involve epidermis, dermis, subcutaneous tissue and blood vessels. Flaps are selected when an area of full-thickness tissue loss occurs. The flap can be completely removed from the donor area and applied to a recipient area, where the blood vessels will be anastamosed to ensure viability of the flap — this can be referred to as a free island flap. Another method of flap is a rotational flap, where an area of tissue can be lifted and rotated to cover a defect which is in close proximity, but where the blood supply is still maintained.

Table 2.5: Principles of management of surgical wounds

- There are many varied surgical techniques that can result in the development of a wound: incisions or excisions, investigative or corrective, open or keyhole

- Four types of wound healing are generally recognised: primary closure, healing by first intention; open granulation, healing by secondary intention; delayed or secondary closure, sometimes called healing by third intention or tertiary intention; and grafting or flap formation

- The two main potential complications following surgical intervention are infection and dehiscence

- Early identification of surgical wound infection can reduce the damage to the wound

- The aim for all surgical wounds is to provide an optimal wound healing environment, which involves minimal disturbance to the wound and the prevention of bacterial invasion

---

Surgical wound complications

The two main complications following surgical intervention are infection and dehiscence. Early signs of wound infection are defined by redness, pain, heat and swelling of the wound and peri-wound area. These signs must not be confused with the inflammatory stage of wound healing, around days three to seven post-operatively.

Infection, among other contributing factors, can lead to dehiscence of the surgical wound: where the wound either partially or fully opens following primary closure. The options following dehiscence are to allow the wound to heal by secondary intention or by delayed closure.

Post-operative wound care will vary from centre to centre and practitioner to practitioner. However, the treatment aims for all surgical wounds are to provide an optimal wound healing environment, which involves minimal disturbance to the wound, and prevention of bacterial invasion.

Traumatic wounds

Skin tears

Skin tears usually occur in the elderly, or individuals with friable skin, and are often due to underlying medical conditions or long-term use of steroid medications. The trauma is frequently located in the individual's extremities, such as arms and lower leg, where an accidental bump or knock causes a skin tear and the epidermis is displaced but still retains the blood supply.

The most efficient way to manage these wounds is to reapply the skin tear, trying to bring the wound edges together to heal by first intention. This may be achieved by initially moistening the wound to facilitate reapplication of the skin tear. Once reapplied, Steri-Strips™ and/or a non-adhesive dressing can retain the skin tear; this should be secured using an appropriate secondary dressing.

If treated at the time of injury and the skin is reapplied, even with the most friable of skin, good skin cover can be achieved.

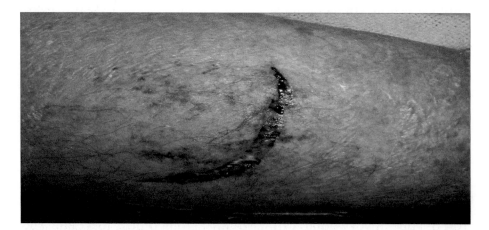

Figure 2.5: Skin tear

Grazes and abrasions

Grazes and abrasions are superficial injuries which are caused by falling onto a rough or gritty surface and the skin is rubbed or torn (Dealey, 1994). They should be cleansed thoroughly to ensure that no foreign bodies remain embedded in the wound bed. Due to the nature of their occurrence, these wounds are often painful.

The majority of these wounds can be effectively treated with a simple, non/low-adherent dressing. However, if painful, the individual may benefit from the application of a film or hydrocolloid dressing, which occludes the wound and keeps the nerve endings moist, therefore reducing the pain. Due to their superficial nature, these wounds should heal quite quickly.

Lacerations

A laceration is a wound caused by blunt trauma, which has split or torn the skin forming jagged wound edges (Collins *et al*, 2002). A thorough assessment of the wound should be carried out to ensure that there is no underlying structure trauma. If the wound edges are clean, closure can be obtained by first intention through Steri-Strips™, glue, or suturing (Dealey, 1994). If the wound is contaminated, primary closure is not indicated, and the wound should be treated with a topical antimicrobial until the infection is cleared. The wound should then be encouraged to heal by secondary intention and moist wound management.

Penetrating and stab wounds

Knives, bullets or other sharp missiles may cause penetrating wounds (Thomas, 1990). Although the external appearance of a penetrating wound may suggest that the injury is relatively minor, internal damage can be considerable, depending upon the site and depth of the penetration, and/or the velocity of the bullet or missile (Owen-Smith, 1985). Prior to implementing any treatment plan, the wound should be thoroughly explored by a doctor as surgery may be necessary.

Table 2.6: Principles of management of traumatic wounds

- Identify and, if appropriate, remove the source of trauma

- If the wound is contaminated or debris is present, ensure that it is cleansed thoroughly

- Thorough assessment should be carried out to ascertain if there is any underlying structure trauma

- Treat the wound following the principles of the Wound Healing Continuum, based on accurate classification and wound assessment

- Always document plan of care and action taken in the individual's care records

Burns

Burns require separate consideration from other traumatic wounds, due to the specialised nature of care required for their treatment. The following show the varying forms of burns.

- **Thermal burns:** these can either be caused by dry heat, such as fires, flash flames, friction, or by wet heat, usually referred to as scalds from hot liquid.

- **Chemical burns:** these involve chemicals of an acid or alkaline nature.

- **Electrical burns:** these can be low voltage, usually a domestic accident <1,000 volts. High voltage burns are industrial accidents, often involving power lines, >1,000 volts.

- **Radiation burns:** these are caused by accidental exposure to ultra-violet light, x-rays and gamma rays.

Extent of burns

The extent of a burn is described by a percentage that indicates the amount of the total body surface area (TBSA) involved. There is little consensus to determine what constitutes a minor scald, which can be treated as an outpatient, and what TBSA should be involved before a referral to a specialist centre is made (Fowler, 1999). Young patients with 5%–10% TBSA should be referred to a specialist centre along with adults who have 5%–10% burns to their face and hands (Turner, 1998). Any individual with 10% or more of the TBSA as a superficial partial-thickness burn would benefit from a review at a specialist centre.

Burn classifications

The depth of tissue penetrated by the thermal insult determines the classification of the burn. The various levels of severity are:

❖ **Superficial burns:** these only involve the epidermis. The skin is dry and intact, but very red and painful to touch. They may form blisters but will usually heal within three to seven days, with minimal or no treatment depending on the formation of the blister (Fowler, 1999). If the skin is intact, it may help to apply a bland moisturiser, or after-sun, to keep the skin supple and rehydrated.

❖ **Superficial partial-thickness burns:** these involve the epidermis and the superficial layer of the dermis. The skin usually shows immediate blistering, is moist and exudes haemoserous fluid. These burns are very painful for the individual (Fowler, 1999). Treatment will require debridement of the blistered areas using a conservative sharp debridement technique. If the wound was contaminated at time of injury, treatment with a topical antimicrobial would be recommended to prevent complications from infection. If the wound is clean, limit dressing changes by applying an absorbent non-adherent dressing, but also ensure that it does not incapacitate the individual's ability to move and exercise the affected area.

❖ **Deep partial-thickness, deep dermal burns:** these are burns which involve the epidermis and dermis, but leave the hair follicles and sebaceous glands intact (Fowler, 1999). The burn appears as white/creamy in colour, with blistering. They can be treated by either debridement and grafting, or, if the area is small, autolytic debridement of the burn tissue, and active treatment with moist dressings.

❖ **Full-thickness burns**: these involve all structural layers: epidermis, dermis, subcutaneous layer and/or deeper structures. The appearance of the skin is one of a waxy-white, grey area or yellow/black translucent leathery appearance (Fowler, 1999). Due to the damage of the nerve endings there is little pain associated with these wounds, but wound edges can be sensitive. These wounds require surgical intervention with extensive debridement and grafting.

Complex wounds

The title complex wounds refers to wounds which may have an underlying pathophysiology, eg. *pyoderma gangrenosum*, necrotising fasciitis, or where wounds may be complicated by the individual's prevalent medical condition, such as rheumatoid arthritis. It is beyond the scope of this chapter to discuss all of these types of wounds, however, the following will be discussed:

- *pyoderma gangrenosum*
- necrotising fasciitis
- fungating tumours.

Pyoderma gangrenosum

Pyoderma gangrenosum is an immunologically-mediated chronic necrotising ulcerative cutaneous condition of the skin (Powell and Perry, 1996). *Pyoderma gangrenosum* often affects a person with an underlying internal disease such as:

- inflammatory bowel diseases (ulcerative colitis and Crohn's disease)
- rheumatoid arthritis
- chronic active hepatitis
- tumours (solid) (Gudi *et al*, 2000).

Pyoderma gangrenosum usually starts quite suddenly, often at the site of a minor injury, and mainly affects the legs and feet (von den Driesch,

1997). It may start as a small pustule, red bump, or blood-blister. The skin then breaks down resulting in an ulcer. The ulcer can deepen and widen rapidly. Characteristically, the edge of the ulcer is purple and undermined as it enlarges. It is usually very painful. Several ulcers may develop at the same time. Left untreated, the ulcers may continue to enlarge, persist unchanged, or may slowly heal.

Treatment with oral or topical steroids is usually successful in arresting the process, but complete healing may take months. Modern moist wound healing products may play a role in promoting healing if the individual is commenced on oral steroids. Patients with *pyoderma gangrenosum* are normally cared for by a dermatologist.

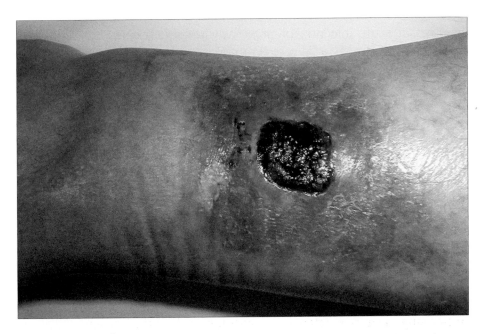

Figure 2.6: *Pyoderma gangrenosum*

Necrotising fasciitis

Necrotising fasciitis is a relatively rare, life-threatening condition, where bacterial toxins invade and destroy large areas of tissue. The most common bacteria associated with necrotising fasciitis is the group A haemolytic streptoccous, commonly known as *Streptococcus pyogenes*. It may enter the body through a long-standing chronic wound, or through an acute wound entry site (Timmons, 2005). Diagnosis can be difficult. The following clinical features are linked with necrotising fasciitis:

- rapid progression
- poor therapeutic response
- blistering necrosis
- cyanosis
- localised tenderness
- pyrexia
- tachycardia
- hypotension
- altered level of consciousness.

In cases of acute infection of previously unbroken skin, the time from injury to development of severe symptoms can be very short (0–2 hours).

Clinically, it often starts with pain — this may be increased pain if the wound already exists. The pain then changes to swelling and soft tissue erythema that does not respond to antibiotics. There is a rapid progression to a grey/blue skin followed by necrosis (Timmons, 2005).

Treatment

Intravenous antibiotics should be administered as soon as possible in an attempt to slow down the invading bacteria.

Aggressive surgical debridement is essential, with the removal of all non-viable tissue with a wide margin. This is to try and prevent recurrence.

Fungating tumours

Fungating wounds arise as the tumour infiltrates the skin and its supporting blood and lymphatic vessels. Unless the malignant cells are checked, the fungation extends and has the potential to cause massive damage to the wound through a combination of rapid growth, loss of vascularity, and ulceration and necrosis (Grocott, 2000).

The management of these wounds is complex, based on a balance between symptom control and patient comfort and acceptability. A great many decisions are reached as a result of information provided by the individual; what they are experiencing and their concerns. Issues relating to pain, odour and exudate are frequently raised, and these should be prioritised when assessing and implementing care.

Table 2.7: Principles of management of complex wounds
• Rapid diagnosis and specialist referral
• Always establish the underlying pathology of the wound
• Recognise the impact that underlying conditions such as rheumatoid arthritis might have
• Seek specialist advice or referral to ensure that the underlying pathology is managed effectively

These types of wound are an example of where an underlying condition can result in the development of a wound: emphasising the need to identify the factors that have led to the development of the wound. Where a wound cannot be identified as fitting into the first five categories, it can be categorised as a complex wound and consideration should be given to the need for specialist referral/advice. Wounds, such as fungating lesions, vasculitic ulcers, or those of unknown pathology, are other examples of complex wounds.

Conclusion

The management of wounds is based on an understanding of the wound's aetiology, any underlying pathophysiology, a full assessment and then appropriate treatment interventions. This chapter provides an overview of some of the common wound types and highlights their key management principles.

References

Allman RM (1997) Pressure ulcer prevalence, incidence, risk factors and impact. *Clin Geriatric Med* **13**(3): 421–36

Baxter H (2003) Management of surgical wounds. *Nurs Times* **99**(13): 66–8

Benbow SJ, Cossins L, MacFarlane IA (1999) Painful diabetic neuropathy. *Diabetic Med* **16**: 632–44

Benbow SJ, Daousi C, MacFarlane IA (2004) Diagnosing and managing chronic painful diabetic neuropathy. *The Diabetic Foot* **7**(1): 34–44

Berg RW (1986) Etiology and pathophysiology of diameter dermatitis. *Adv Dermatol* **3**: 102–6

Bliss M (1990) (Editorial) Preventing pressure sores. *Lancet* **335**: 1311–12

Bianchi J (2005) LOI: an alternative to Doppler in leg ulcer patients. *Wounds UK* **1**(1): 80–5

Bonham P (2003) Assessment and management of patients with venous, arterial, and diabetic/neuropathic lower extremity wounds. *Am Association of Critical Care Nurses* **14**(4): 442–56

Browse NL, Burns KG, Lea Thomas M (1988) *Diseases of the Veins: pathology, diagnosis and treatment*. Edward Arnold, London

Cawley MI (1987) Vasculitis and ulceration in rheumatic diseases of the foot. *Baillieres Clin Rheumatol* **1**(2): 315–33

Cullum N, Roe B (1995) *Leg Ulcers Nursing Management — a research-based guide*. Baillière Tindall, London

Cooper P, Russell F, Stringfellow SA (2004) A review of different wound types and their principles of management. *Applied Wound Management Supplement I*. Wounds UK, Aberdeen

Cornwall J, Dore CJ, Lewis JD (1986) Leg ulcers: epidemiology and aetiology. *Br J Surg* **73**: 693–6

Dormandy JA, Murray GD (1991) The fate of the claudicant: a prospective study of 1969 claudicants. *Eur J Vasc Surg* **5**: 131–3

Dealey C (1994) *The Care of Wounds*. Blackwell Science, Oxford

De P, Kunze G, Gibby OM, Harding K (2000) Outcome of diabetic foot ulcers in a specialist foot clinic. *The Diabetic Foot* **4**(3): 131–6

Defloor T, Grypdonck MHF (1999) Sitting posture and prevention of pressure ulcers. *Appl Nurs Res* **12**(3): 136–42

European Pressure Ulcer Advisory Panel (2002) Guide to pressure ulcer grading. *EPUAP Review* **3**(3): 75

Fiers SA (1996) Breaking the cycle: The etiology of incontinence dermatitis and evaluating and using skin care products. *Ostomy Wound Management* **42**(3): 33–43

Foster A, Edmons ME (1987) Examination of the diabetic foot. _Practical Diabetes_ 4(3): 105–6

Fowler A (1999) Burns. In: Miller M, Glover D, eds. _Wound Management Theory and Practice_. Nursing Times Books, London

Gebhardt K, Bliss MR (1994) Preventing pressure sores in orthopedic patients — is prolonged chair nursing detrimental? _J Tissue Viability_ 4(2): 51–4

Gosnell D (1973) An assessment tool to identify pressure sores. _Nurs Residential Care_ **22**: 55–9

Gray D, White RJ, Cooper P (2003) The wound healing continuum. In: White RJ, ed. _The Silver Book_. Quay Books, MA Healthcare Ltd, London

Gray D, Cooper P, Clark M (1999) Pressure ulcer prevention in an acute hospital. Poster presentation, EPUAP, Amsterdam 1999

Grocott P (2000) The palliative management of fungating malignant wounds. _J Wound Care_ **9**(1): 4–9

Gudi VS, Julian C, Bowers PW (2000) Pyoderma gangrenosum complicating bilateral mammoplasty. _Br J Plastic Surg_ **53**: 440–1

Günnewicht B, Dunford C (2004) _Fundamental Aspects of Tissue Viability Nursing_. Quay Books, MA Healthcare Ltd, London

Hurst RT, Lee RW (2003) Increased incidence of coronary artherosclerosis in type 2 diabetes mellitus: mechanisms and management. _Ann Intern Med_ **139**: 824–34

Jones J (2000) The use of holistic assessment in the treatment of leg ulcers. _Br J Nurs_ **9**(16): 1040–52

Jordan MM, Clark M, Barbanel CL _et al_ (1977) Incidence of pressure sores in the Greater Glasgow Health Board area. _Lancet_ **2**: 548–50

Leyden JJ, Katz S, Stewart R, Kligman AM (1977) Urinary ammonia and ammonia producing micro-organisms in infants with and without diaper dermatitis. _Arch Dermatol_ **113**: 1678–80

Krentz AM, Acheson P, Basu A, Kilvert A, Wright AD, Nattrass M (1997) Morbidity and mortality associated with diabetic foot disease: a 12-month prospective survey of hospital admissions in a single UK centre. _Foot_ **7**: 144–7

Maklebust J (1987) Pressure ulcers, aetiology and prevention. _Nurs Clin North Am_ **22**(2): 359–77

Morison M, Moffat C (1994) _A Colour Guide to the Assessment and Management of Leg Ulcers_. Mosby, St Louis

Nelzen O, Bergqvist D, Lindhagen A (1993) High prevalence of diabetes in chronic leg ulcer patients: a cross-sectional population study. _Diabet Med_ **10**: 345–50

NHS Quality Improvement (2003) _Best Practice Statement for the Prevention of Pressure Ulcers_. NHS Quality Improvement, Scotland

Norton D, McLaren R, Exton-Smith A (1962) *An Investigation of Geriatric Nursing Problems in Hospital*. Churchill Livingstone, Edinburgh

Owen-Smith M (1985) Wounds caused by the weapons of war. In: Westaby S, ed. *Wound Care*. Heinemann Medical, London: 110–20

Powell FC, Su WP, Perry HO (1996) Pyoderma gangrenosum: classification and management. *J Am Acad Dermatol* **34**: 395–409

Pudner R (1998) The management of patients with a leg ulcer. *J Community Nurs* **12**(5): 26–33

Royal College of Nursing (1998) *Clinical Practice Guidelines: The Management of Patients with Venous Leg Ulcers*. RCN Institute, Centre for Evidence-Based Nursing, University of York and the School of Nursing, Midwifery and Health Visiting, University of Manchester

Rycroft-Malone J (2000) *Clinical Practice Guidelines. Pressure Ulcer Risk Assessment and Prevention*. RCN, London

Scottish Intercollegiate Guidelines Network (1998) *The Care of Patients with Chronic Leg Ulcers*. SIGN, Edinburgh

Shearman CP, Chulakadabba A (1999) The value of risk factor management in patients with peripheral arterial disease. In: *The Evidence for Vascular Surgery*. Tfm Publishing, Harley, Shropshire

Sumner DS (1989) Non-invasive assessment of peripheral arterial occlusive disease. In: Rutherford KS, ed. *Vascular Surgery*. 3rd edn. WB Saunders, Philadelphia

Thomas S (1990) *Wound Management and Dressings*. The Pharmaceutical Press, London

Timmons J (2005) Recognising fasciitis. *Wounds UK* **1**(2): 40–5

Torrance C (1983) *Pressure Sore: Aetiology, treatment and prevention*. Croom Helm, London

Towey AP, Erland SM (1988) Validity and reliability of an assessment tool for pressure ulcer risk. *Decubitus* **1**(2): 40–2

Turner DG (1998) Ambulatory care of the burn patient. In: Carrougher GJ, ed. *Burn Care and Therapy*. Mosby, St Louis

von den Driech P (1997) Pyoderma gangrenosum: a report of 44 cases with follow-up. *Br J Dermatol* **137**: 1000–5

Waterlow J (1985) A risk assessment card. *Nurs Times* **81**(48): 49–55

Wounds UK (2005) *Best Practice Statement for Compression Hosiery*. Wounds UK, Aberdeen

Young T (2004) The 30-degree tilt vs the 90-degree lateral and supine positions in reducing the incidence of non-blanching erythema in a hospital inpatient population: a randomised controlled trial. *J Tissue Viability* **14**(3): 88, 90, 92–6

Self-assessment exercises

Consider the following patient.

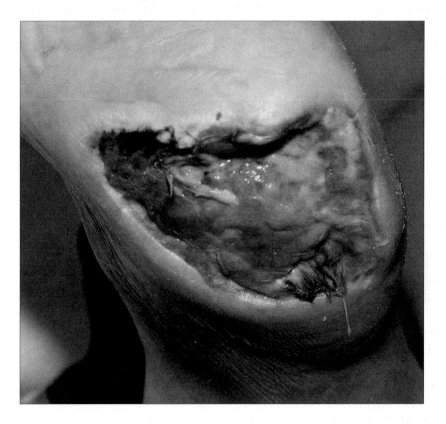

What type of chronic wound is shown here?

What are the potential causes of this wound?

What would your treatment of a patient with this type of wound involve?

What additional factors should be considered when treating this patient?

Study the photograph below and identify, first, the type of wound, and then describe how you would assess this patient?

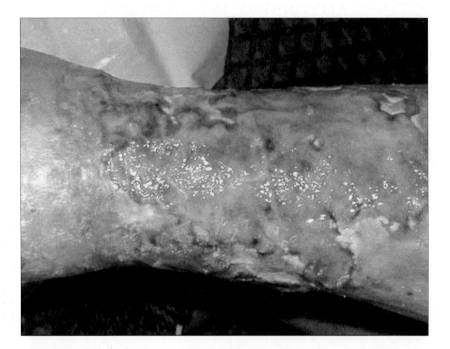

Consider a patient that you have cared for with a complex wound.

How did you assess this patient?

Given the information within this chapter, how will your patient assessment change?

CHAPTER 3

FACTORS ADVERSELY INFLUENCING WOUND HEALING

John Timmons

Introduction

This chapter highlights a number of systemic and social factors that may significantly influence wound healing. Assessment of these factors is considered in a holistic context that extends beyond the familiar review of the wound site, to include chronic illnesses and the prevailing social circumstances.

It is important that staff attending to patients' wounds are aware of the factors influencing healing, as these impinge on wound assessment and the prescribing of wound care products.

There are a number of convenient but not so helpful assumptions made about patients and their wounds. The first of these is that wound care can be separated in some practical way from the circumstances of the patient. There exists substantial literature on wound healing, dressings and treatments designed to enhance or speed up the healing process. Research evidence offered about the efficacy of different dressings and findings, usually ignores the influence of systemic and social or environmental factors upon the healing process. It is extremely easy to become focused on the changes underway at the wound site. The second, and rather paradoxical assumption, is that nurses assess patients in a holistic way. We nurse the 'whole person' and are encouraged to see individuals in their social contexts. This begs the question: How can we arrange an assessment approach that adequately explores the ways in which factors influence wound healing at different levels?

Acute wounds are wounds that generally progress in the desired fashion; that is, they can be seen to move through the identified stages towards healing. Acute wounds include abrasions, lacerations, minor burns and surgical wounds healing through primary intention. Chronic wounds, however, do not progress swiftly towards healing. It is generally accepted that if a wound has not healed within six weeks, it may be considered to be a chronic wound (Kane and Krasner, 1997). Chronic wounds include pressure ulcers, leg ulcers, deep burns and may include surgical wounds left to heal through secondary intention.

To ensure holistic treatment we must employ an assessment tool that encourages the nurse to examine the ways in which factors interact either to promote or to undermine wound healing (*Figure 3.1*). While at this stage research evidence is neither detailed nor complete enough to help us quantify the risk value for each factor, the idea of weighing risks remains important. Nursing models encourage such holistic assessment. It is useful for nurses to appreciate the ways in which risk factors in different zones may accumulate to undermine wound healing. By making observations and creating records that relate to each of the patient's key problems, we will be in a better position to appreciate where to lay the emphasis of care, and when to consider an alternative environment within which wound healing might be facilitated.

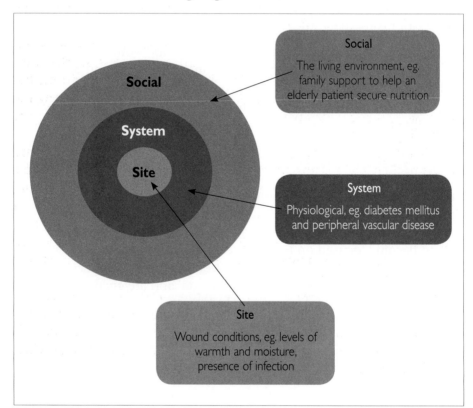

Figure 3.1: Zonal influences on wound healing (adapted from Timmons, 2003)

Risk factors accumulate at the systemic and social level, and may prove powerful enough to undermine the use of dressings or treatments employed at the wound site, regardless of how advanced the therapy may be.

This happens in a number of ways, such as:

- by undermining the volume or the quality of support available to the patient as he or she tries to self-care and reduce the risk of further damage to the wound
- by damaging the physiological environment required to promote wound healing (eg. supply of blood to the wound site)
- by increasing the chances of interference to wound healing measures (eg. when a confused patient interferes with wound dressings).

Risk factors identified at these levels might either prompt direct action by the nurse (for instance, to improve nutrition), or adjustments in the care of the wound site itself (for instance, selecting a dressing that minimises the risk of introducing infection).

The healing process entails a complex and dynamic series of activities at a vascular and cellular level. For healing to progress satisfactorily, these processes need to be controlled. If they are disrupted during the inflammatory phase (which initiates the healing cascade), or during the proliferative phase (when new tissue is being generated), this will impede the healing process.

Inflammatory responses to injury that occur early on include release of neutrophils and plasma proteins from the blood to the extracellular fluid. The neutrophils are actively involved in wound cleansing, keeping the wound free of debris and bacteria by phagocytic activity. The plasma proteins additionally initiate and accelerate the inflammatory response. Examples will be given later on as to how alterations in biology, the care delivered, and environmental issues can lead to factors that negatively influence wound healing.

Factors may be viewed as being either intrinsic (ie. emanating from within the patient), or extrinsic (ie. external to the patient). Occasionally, confusion may arise when it is difficult to identify clearly whether a factor is intrinsic or extrinsic in origin, such as when considering nutrition or drugs.

Intrinsic factors

The intrinsic factors presented here are:

- circulatory insufficiency
- the ageing patient
- body build
- chronic wound exudate
- the importance of nutritional status in wound healing
- concurrent illness
- diabetes
- renal disease
- rheumatoid arthritis
- psychosocial factors.

Circulatory insufficiency

Insufficient blood supply could potentially lead to a decrease in the oxygen and nutrients delivered to the tissues, which could delay wound healing and have an impact on local healthy tissue.

Some examples of concurrent illness which may lead to a reduced blood supply are:

- cardiovascular disease
- anaemia
- haemorrhage
- respiratory disease
- peripheral vascular disease (PVD).

All cells require the regular supply of oxygen and nutrients to ensure cell function, growth and division. Consider then the impact of conditions which affect the delivery of key nutrients to local tissues. Not only will delayed healing result, but the presence of some conditions will actually predispose the patient to the development of wounds, such as leg ulcers. Anaemia, for example, irrespective of the cause, will result in reduced oxygen-carrying capacity of the blood.

It is known that collagen synthesis (which is essential to prevent pressure damage) is reliant on the supply of oxygen and nutrients, including vitamin C. A reduction in the availability of these components may be implicated in a loss of tensile strength of the scar during wound healing (Kanzler *et al*, 1986). Re-injury at a later date is therefore a risk. The risk of wound infection also increases in tissue hypoxia. Neutrophils and other white cells responsible for phagocytosis (engulfing bacteria), will not function in an oxygen-poor environment.

It is important to consider this when deciding on the optimal treatment regime for patient groups where concurrent illnesses are present.

The ageing patient

The process of ageing represents both social and physical risks. Ageing involves facing social, psychological and physiological challenges (*Table 3.1*). The UK has one of the demographically oldest populations within Europe (Kinsella, 1996). It is estimated that by 2021 there will be almost sixty people of pensionable age per hundred people of working age (Office of Population Census and Surveys [OPCS], 1996). The resultant rise in elderly patient numbers could bring with it an increased risk of chronic and/or non-healing wounds. Social and system changes combine to complicate both the assessment and the management of wounds.

To understand this better, it is useful to study the factors which age the human body. Kyriazis (1994) believed that although many theories of ageing are inconclusive, they fall into two main camps, namely:

❖   Theories which believe that ageing is caused by factors that can lead to damage to the body, such as toxic by-products of metabolism, everyday damage, radiation and genes that are known to promote ageing.
❖   Theories which point to the damage being poorly repaired due to a lack of metabolic energy, hormone deficiency, immune system failure, to name but a few.

Regardless of which theory is 'correct', the result for the ageing person can be seen in prolonged periods of ill health and a slower response to injury.

Age-related changes within the body are most apparent with changes in the skin; therefore, it is easy to understand the impact that such changes can have on wound healing (Ford and Willis, 2002). The changes in the skin include thinning, a loss of elasticity due to collagen depletion, and reduction in the blood and nerve supply. Skin pigmentation also changes, atrophy of sweat glands occurs, and reduced sebum production causes the skin to appear dry and flaky.

The patient is less likely to respond to pain stimuli and, therefore, injury may incur more frequently with wounds being slower to heal. The loss of collagen from the skin also makes the patient more vulnerable to pressure damage.

Of course, the ageing process will affect more than the skin of the patient and changes can be noted in all of the body's systems (*Figure 3.2*).

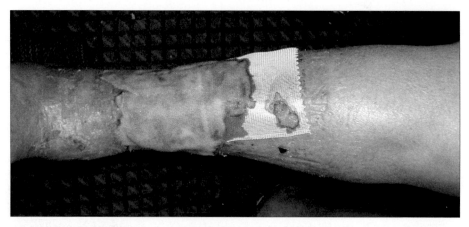

Figure 3.2: Leg ulcer on an eighty-nine-year-old lady with venous disease, chronic obstructive pulmonary disease and arthritis

Body build

Obesity

Obesity is considered a risk factor in many areas of practice, no less in wound management. The person suffering from obesity is more likely to have reduced mobility, increasing the risk of pressure sore development and the subsequent formation of chronic wounds, such as pressure and leg ulcers.

Table 3.1: Social and systemic threats to wound healing associated with ageing

Social threats	
Comparative isolation	In extreme old age there is a significant reduction in the number of friends and family available to help the patient sustain self-care
Housing conditions	Living conditions of the elderly may be poor with increased risk of injury
Social disengagement	After retirement, there are fewer opportunities to engage with others or opportunities for others to help identify developing problems
Psychological system changes	
Changes to self-esteem	Faced with deteriorating body functions, the elderly person may doubt his or her ability to change circumstances or solve problems
Mood changes	Social isolation and the challenges of dealing with multiple health problems undermine morale and may lead to depression, aggression or withdrawal
Self-care standards	The elderly person loses the volition to sustain standards of self-care, and body image is undermined by accumulating physical changes (see below)
Physiological system changes	
Neurological changes	Reactions become slower due to the decrease in the number of synapse axions
Cardiopulmonary system	Cardiac output drops due to fibrosis and sclerosis in the endocardium. The heart rate slows and there is decreased pulmonary efficiency with increased risk of bacterial growth
Gastrointestinal system	Patients eat smaller, more frequent meals because of a reduction in gastric secretion. Decreased taste buds may cause a subsequent reduction in appetite. The elderly person may be prone to constipation
Musculoskeletal system	Loss of subcutaneous tissue may increase susceptibility to pressure damage. Bone degeneration and reduced joint flexibility occur
Endocrine system	Glucose tolerance and the ability to thermoregulate decrease
Special senses	Sense of smell and taste decrease. There is a reduction in visual acuity and hearing diminishes
Kidneys and genitourinary system	Due to a decrease in renal blood flow, there is a reduction in the glomerular filtration rate. A decrease in bladder size and loss of sphincter control may also occur. In males, the prostate may enlarge. In females, oestrogen levels are reduced and there is a decrease in lubrication of the female genital tract

In many studies (Kozol *et al*, 1986; Perkins, 1992), it has been shown that patients who are overweight are more likely to suffer wound healing problems in the post-operative phase due to a lack of oxygen in the tissues. This results in a reduction in the amount of collagen produced, reducing the tensile strength of the wound (Kozol *et al*, 1986).

Tissue bulk increases tension on tissues, and the risk of dehiscence (Perkins, 1992) and hernia formation increases accordingly. Haematoma formation is also more likely in obese patients (Kozol *et al*, 1986). With seromas, raised pressures within a wound impede the oxygen supply to the tissues and delay healing.

Patients suffering from obesity may also suffer from accompanying medical problems such as diabetes, cardiopulmonary and vascular disorders; all of which can have an adverse effect on wound healing as healing tissues rely on an optimal supply of oxygen (see 'Circulatory insufficiency', p. 50).

One common mistake in treating wounds in this patient group is to assume that they are well-nourished. This may not be the case, and it is still necessary to give nutritional supplements which can help to support the wound healing process and prevent complications.

The thin patient

Many patients with wounds may present in a state of cachexia or in a 'catabolic' state. When the body suffers stress its energy stores are used up to supply existing demands, resulting in loss of weight. Protein-energy malnutrition is a term that is used to describe a reduction in macronutrients and many micronutrients.

Without key proteins and essential nutrients there is inadequate synthesis of collagen and a consequent delay in healing. There is also little energy to help fuel the wound healing process.

The patient will also be at risk of pressure ulcer development from the loss of tissue over bony prominences.

Chronic wound exudate

Chronic wounds often produce exudate which is not only copious, but also known to be damaging to the essential growth factors and the extracellular matrix (ECM). Wounds subsequently fail to re-epithelialise and the inflammatory response is prolonged (Thomas, 2001). The amount of exudate, if uncontrolled, can contribute to maceration of the surrounding skin and, ultimately, lead to extension of the wound itself (Miller and Dyson, 1996).

Exudate from chronic wounds has been shown to slow down or stop the proliferation of key cells such as keratinocytes, fibroblasts and endothelial cells (Vowden *et al*, 2002). Chronic wound exudate contains excess proteinase, which is known to break down peptide links within the growth factors, and also to affect the build up of the ECM. As the ECM is essential for the laying down of new cells and capillaries, any disruption to this stage prolongs healing. The proteases responsible for this are the matrix metalloproteinases (MMPs). MMPs play an important role in cell migration and in re-modelling of the wound post injury. However, in chronic wounds, the large numbers being produced in the exudate can have a negative impact on healing (Parks, 1999).

Moore (2003) cited the key issues of exudate in chronic wound healing as having an inhibitory effect on:

- endothelial proliferation
- fibroblast proliferation
- keratinocyte proliferation
- collagen synthesis.

The proteases may also degrade growth factors and ECM components.

With this in mind, treatment of excess exudate in chronic wounds should be two-fold, both direct and indirect (Vowden et al, 2002).

❖ Direct treatments involve measures to help reduce the level of exudate, by simple absorption using absorbent foam dressings. Compression therapy and topical negative pressure, such as the VAC® system, may also be used to address oedema in venous disease of the lower limbs (Mendez–Eastman, 1998).

❖ Indirect methods address the problems which cause excess exudate production, such as infection or bacterial load. Key products to reduce bacteria in the wound include cadexomer iodine and those containing silver (Falanga, 1999; Cutting and White 2002).

Systemic treatment of heart failure may also help to reduce oedema in limbs. Reducing the extracellular fluid present in the tissues therefore helps to reduce local wound exudate.

Recently, the role of freeze-dried bovine collagen has been effective in reducing the action of wound proteases, such as MMPs. The product has been shown to have a number of modes of action specific to non-healing chronic wounds (Cullen *et al*, 2002). The resultant reduction in protease activity has a direct effect on wound healing by allowing the ECM to form in the normal way (Cullen *et al*, 2002). In addition to its action on protease activity, the product also binds the growth factors present to protect them and then release them in a bioactive form (Moore, 2003). Fibroblast migration has also been shown to increase under the action of this product, thus effectively speeding up the healing process (Hart *et al*, 2002).

Freeze-dried bovine collagen has been tested on a variety of compromised wounds and been effective in treating venous leg ulcers and diabetic foot ulceration (Hart *et al*, 2002).

The importance of nutrition in wound healing

The role of nutrition in wound healing and in general patient well-being is well-documented. Despite this, a number of studies show that many patients in both community and hospital settings remain in an under-nourished state (Martin, 1998; Sitton-Kent and Gilchrist, 1993).

These studies highlight a clear correlation between slow wound healing and sub-clinical malnutrition. Of fifty-nine patients within a community trust with chronic wounds, the majority of cases had a level of sub-clinical malnutrition (Martin, 1998).

The wound healing process is complex, requiring a number of nutritional factors to be present to meet the demands that the wound is making on the patient (Gray and Cooper, 2001). During the process of healing, the metabolic rate increases, as does cellular activity. Adenosine triphosphate provides the energy for this activity by its synthesis from glucose, which is a by-product of carbohydrate metabolism. As an energy source, carbohydrates are key to the process.

Nutritional status

The ingestion of 'calories', usually measured as kilocalories and abbreviated to kcal, is commonly associated with dieting and weight loss. A wound makes heavy demands on stored energy. Approximately 2500 kcal/

day are required to heal a moderately-sized wound. This increases to 4,000–4,500 kcal/day in large wounds that have become infected, so that enough energy is present for the formation of antibodies, collagen, fibroblasts, white blood cells and angiogenesis. One gram of protein or carbohydrate provides 4.6 kcal of energy, and one gram of fat generates 9.2 kcal.

When considering nutrition and wound healing:

- carbohydrates are required for cellular activity, proliferation and phagocytic activity
- fats are required to provide energy and maintain cell membrane
- protein is required for repair and generation of connective tissue, blood vessels, and new epithelium.

Malnutrition increases the risk of wound infection as these patients have an impaired immune response (Olde Damink and Soeters, 1997).

It is important that water is not omitted from 'nutrition'. Although water is not a nutrient, it is essential to avoid dehydration as this will affect cellular metabolism and circulating volume and oxygen delivery.

Proteins are necessary for the inflammatory phase of healing, both for new cell growth and, in particular, collagen is synthesised from amino acids taken from protein intake. Protein depletion has been linked to slow healing and may lead to weaker scar formation.

Fat is also required as many fatty acids cannot be synthesised by the body; it is believed that these are involved in cell membrane formation (Lewis and Harding, 1993).

Other key nutritional elements needed for wound healing include vitamins, trace elements and minerals (Gray *et al*, 2001).

Poor nutritional state has also been linked to an increased risk of pressure ulcer development in patients within nursing homes (Pinchcofski-Devin and Kaminski, 1986).

In practice, it is essential that we properly assess patients' nutritional status as well as assessing their wounds. The implementation of a wound assessment chart may be necessary to allow continuity of documentation and approach to patient care. The simplest method of improving nutritional status is merely convincing the patient to eat more, however, if this is not possible, the provision of nutritional supplements, enteral and/or parenteral, may be necessary (Lennard-Jones, 1992)

Concurrent illness

Concurrent illness will place demands on the resources that would in other circumstances be directed to support the healing process, eg. nutrition and the immune system. Conflict in these demands will result in delays to the healing process.

For example, in patients with malignancy, weight loss may be accompanied by anorexia, weakness and malnutrition. There is also evidence that cancer cells produce plasminogen activators (PA). These activators have been found at the wound edge and floor of leg ulcers, and it is likely that plasminogen activators encourage the migration of keratinocytes, which also secrete PA (Lotti *et al*, 1998).

Diabetes and cardiovascular disease will adversely affect the delivery of oxygen and nutrients to the wound.

Patients who are immunosuppressed may also exhibit slow wound healing due to the failure of what is seen as the 'normal response' to injury.

Key cells involved in the immune response include neutrophils, later followed by macrophages. These cells play an active and vital part during the early stages of healing by keeping the wound clean of debris and countering any potential infection through phagocytic activity.

Diabetes

While diabetes mellitus is the quintessential physiological homeostasis problem, it can also be conceived of in social terms. The diagnosis of this condition brings with it necessary adjustments to diet and skin care, especially the feet. Many patients have difficulty in sustaining these adjustments in their lifestyle. Diabetes mellitus is associated with a number of complicating factors which can lead both to ulceration of the lower limbs and, consequently, poor healing of the resultant wound (Mani *et al*, 1999).

Wounds in patients with diabetes often develop into a chronic or long-standing problem, which becomes difficult to heal for a number of reasons. Raised blood glucose levels may precipitate infection in an open wound, and compromised vascular networks can prevent adequate blood supply and, therefore, slow healing. In addition, the very nature of the chronic or non-healing wound, as they are often referred to, contains a number of inherent characteristics which prevent or prolong the healing process, such as the presence of proteases which are known to break down the extracellular matrix (Falanga, 2000).

Patients with diabetes are likely to develop ulceration as a result of the long-term complications of diabetes. Ulceration is most likely to occur when there is tissue ischaemia and/or in the presence of neuropathy (Newton _et al_, 2001). Ischaemia is normally the result of long-standing damage to the large and small blood vessels of the legs and feet. The resultant damage to the microcirculation can precipitate ulceration but is not directly indicative. The most likely cause of ulceration would be trauma to the area, or skin infection. These events would normally lead to an increase in local perfusion, however, if ischaemia exists, this will not take place. Once an ulcer forms, healing becomes difficult due to poor perfusion, and abnormal blood glucose levels may be associated with bacterial growth in the area (Armstrong, 1996).

Neuropathy can exist on two levels in the diabetic patient: autonomic and sensorimotor (Mani _et al_, 1999). In cases where autonomic nerve damage is apparent, there is a loss of muscle tone, alteration in blood supply, and a reduction in sweating. This reduction in sweating may cause cracks to appear on the patient's skin, which can become a focus for infection resulting in ulceration. Sensorimotor neuropathy results in numbness in the feet and, at times, the patient may complain of contact parasthaesia. The loss of the response to pain may lead to unrecognised injury to the foot caused by trauma, burn injury, or continuous pressure from ill-fitting foot wear. The shape of the foot can also change from loss of motor nerve function, creating areas of excess pressure and the potential for ulceration. Continued destruction of the bones and joints in the foot is often referred to as Charcot's foot (Larsen _et al_, 2001).

In some patients, the presence of ischaemia and neuropathy can coexist — 40% of patients with ulceration (Mani _et al_, 1999) — resulting in an adverse prognosis. The key themes for clinical management of these patients are:

- prevention of limb damage through careful screening
- patient education regarding inspection of the feet
- strict control of blood sugar levels.

A multidisciplinary approach is essential in order to give holistic care to this group of patients.

Renal disease

The kidneys are responsible for homeostasis and providing a suitable environment for optimal cellular function through selective excretion and re-absorption (Walsh, 2002). In addition to the excretory function, the kidneys are responsible for the production of rennin, erythropoetin and calcitrol. Patients with renal disease encounter a number of problems because of the complex nature of the role of the kidneys in maintaining the internal environment. The effects of renal disease on wound healing become apparent when examining the far-reaching extent of renal disease. In such patients, the skin is often dry, flaky and the patient may complain of pruritis, which causes the patient to scratch and potentially break the skin.

Wound healing threats associated with renal disease may include:

❖ Protein loss in the urine resulting in oedema, increased risk of blood clotting, raised cholesterol, and an increased risk of infection.
❖ Anaemia caused by decreased production of erythropoetin, resulting in a reduction in the oxygen-carrying capacity of the blood to the area.
❖ Uraemia which can lead to anorexia, nausea and, thus, adversely affect the nutritional state of the patient. The uraemic patient will have clotting problems and bleed easily due to defective platelets.
❖ Peripheral neuropathy may also be present in advanced disease, leading to unintentional injury.
❖ Fluid and electrolyte imbalance which can result in hyperkalaemia, acidosis, hypocalcaemia and oedema, leading to reduced cellular efficiency.

When dealing with renal patients, the aim of management is to provide adequate patient education to prevent injury and to minimise the risks of non-compliance with dietary regimes. Other care aims are more specific and symptom-related, however, it is vital that the impact of renal disease is not underestimated.

Rheumatoid arthritis

Rheumatoid arthritis is an autoimmune disease in which the body mistakes the synovial lining of joints for a foreign antigen, causing a chronic inflammatory process. The disease is most common in women between the ages of thirty and fifty (Spring House Corporation, 1998). As the inflammation spreads, fibrin in the exudate forms a thick membrane of granulation tissue, known as pannus, which grows over the joint surfaces, eroding cartilage, and possibly also destroying bone surfaces. The scar tissue and resulting fibrosis lead to joint deformity and calcification. The process is insidious, and the patient will experience pain and swelling over the joints. Often nodules develop, containing fibrous material and granulation tissue (Byrne, 1999). Reduced mobility and pain can contribute to the risk of pressure sores.

The systemic effects of rheumatoid arthritis are profound, and many patients with this disorder will experience associated weight loss and fatigue; anaemia is also common. Other key systemic problems which affect the wound healing process include, lymphadenopathy, oedema, peripheral neuropathy, muscle wasting, immobility and vasculitis. Again, it is common in this patient group to find wounds which are of a chronic nature, which may contain sloughy tissue and proteolytic enzymes, and are prone to infection.

In some rheumatoid patients, the small vessels that infiltrate the skin as a result of the exaggerated inflammatory response develop into small vasculitic leg ulcers. In time, these small ulcers may become confluent to produce a large ulcerated area. Treatment often involves the use of steroids and/or chemotherapeutic agents (Mani _et al_, 1999) (_Figure 3.3_).

Psychosocial factors

Stress

The impact of psychological stress on the physical system has been the focus of much attention over the years. Stress can adversely affect our immune system, central nervous system, and the endocrine system.

A study by Glaser (1999), focusing on stress and wound healing, demonstrated depletion of pro-inflammatory cytokines in the early stages of healing. Cytokines are important mediators for wound healing.

There is a risk that stimulation of the sympathetic nervous system as a response to stress will lead to vasoconstriction which, in turn, will lead to impaired tissue perfusion with a resultant lack of oxygen and nutrients reaching the wound area.

The effect of such stress can be multiplied if the stress relates to the presence of a disfiguring wound. Rumsey *et al* (2003) examined the psychosocial impact of disfiguring conditions, and concluded that the needs of this patient group were not being met by the healthcare system.

Holden-Lund (1988) found that lowering stress via relaxation techniques 'demonstrated stress-relieving outcomes closely associated with healing'.

Social factors

The gradual reduction in significant family and friends causes elderly patients to become more isolated. This relative solitude may lead to depression or anxiety. This may also be associated with low income, poor housing, and the subsequent risk of hypothermia during cold weather.

There are a growing number of patients who may have wounds as a result of intravenous drug use, for whom the traditional healthcare system is not viewed as 'sufficiently supportive'. This group may be homeless, or lack good housing, and are generally in the lower income bracket. There is a prevalence for this patient group to have inadequate nutrition, and this, combined with poor living conditions and hygiene, adversely impacts on wound healing.

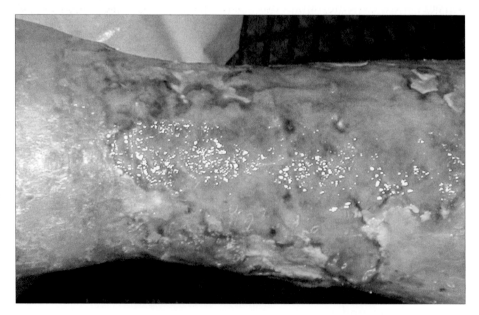

Figure 3.3: Non-healing ulcer in a patient with rheumatoid arthritis

Extrinsic factors

The following are some of the extrinsic factors which may affect the patient.

- drugs
- lifestyle
- infection
- mechanical stress
- temperature
- inappropriate use of antimicrobial agents or dressings
- radiotherapy.

Drugs

Steroid preparations, due to their anti-inflammatory properties, interfere with wound healing. Steroids, non-steroidal anti-inflammatory drugs (NSAIDs), and rheumatoid drugs (also anti-inflammatory) reduce the inflammatory response and, therefore, delay cellular and biochemical activities which initiate the healing process. These products prevent macrophage migration to the site of injury and inhibit the release of collagenase and plasminogen activator (PA). Later on, these products delay fibroblast migration during the reconstructive phase.

Non-steroidals interfere with prostaglandin production, which is a short-lived mediator of inflammatory response and, likewise, delay healing. Cytotoxic drugs delay wound healing by inhibiting cell division and protein synthesis. These agents, used to kill and prevent growth of malignant cells, also interfere with normal cell division. Healthy cellular activity, in the form of proliferation, protein synthesis and a normal inflammatory response, is impeded. The wound cleansing actions are decreased and the risk of infection consequently increased.

Lifestyle

In today's society, it is generally accepted that the lifestyle of many patients may be antagonistic to the aims of the health care which they are receiving. Smoking and alcohol abuse are among the two most damaging 'lifestyle' components which are often viewed as socially acceptable. Alcohol abuse may lead to liver damage, blood clotting problems, and anaemia, as well as malnutrition in many cases (Cutting, 1994).

Tobacco smoke contains over 4000 different compounds or gases. The most well-recognised being nicotine and carbon monoxide. However, many toxic compounds, such as cyanide, heavy metals and other additives, are also present. Both nicotine and carbon monoxide are absorbed quickly into the blood stream. Nicotine causes the release of epinephrine and subsequent vasoconstriction of peripheral vessels, together with an increase in pulse and blood pressure.

Carbon monoxide binds to haemoglobin to form carboxy-haemoglobin, displacing oxygen and making less oxygen available for the tissues. This reduction in the oxygen supply to the tissue is a major impediment to wound healing, particularly in the post-surgical patient (Jensen *et al*, 1991).

It has also been shown that collagen is depleted in smokers, indicating the potential for reduced wound tensile strength and dehiscence in the acute wound (Jorgensen *et al*, 1998)

In one study, four weeks of abstinence from smoking showed a reduction in wound infection as a result of improved neutrophil oxidative killing mechanisms of bacteria (Sorensen *et al*, 2003).

Infection

Bacteria has a variety of effects on wounds. Most chronic wounds will contain levels of bacteria, however, only in some cases will these levels affect the healing process (Dow *et al*, 1999). When the number of bacteria reach sufficient levels and the host response is reduced, infection may occur. Infection may stimulate the release of proteases which break down protein and prolong the the inflammatory phase. Additionally, infection may disrupt clotting mechanisms, impair leucocyte function, increase the size of the wound, and impede epithelialisation. It is important to remember that all chronic wounds are colonised with a plethora of microorganisms.

Dow *et al* (1999) suggested that to detect the bacterial burden one must consider the number and virulence of the bacteria and the host resistance. In some patients who have concurrent illness, the number of bacteria required to affect wound healing is lower than in a healthy host. Similarly, when the strain of the bacteria is particularly virulent, less bacterial presence may impact on wound healing (Sibbald *et al*, 2000). Visual assessment of wounds should be carried out regularly to avoid complications of infection, and to react to tissue changes and slow- or non-healing wounds. Wound swabbing, however, may only be of limited value (Miller *et al*, 1996). Changes that may indicate increased bacterial load include; increase in exudate, abnormal discharge, pain, cellulitis of surrounding tissue, odour, bleeding, and failure to heal (Browne *et al*, 2001). Examining the wound bacteria via swabbing may prove helpful, but to identify correctly bacterial types, tissue sampling may be necessary (Vowden and Vowden, 2002).

Treatment of bacterial burden should focus on removal of dead or necrotic tissue by debridement. In addition, topical antimicrobials may be used to reduce bacterial counts within the wound (Browne *et al*, 2001). Systemic antibiotics are required if the topical treatment fails to have an impact on the wound status, or if there are signs of deeper clinical infection. The dressing regime chosen should reflect the bacterial status of the wound, the exudate level and the odour. Many modern wound dressing products are effective in preventing bacterial transmission through the dressing material, so reducing the risk of cross-infection.

Mechanical stress

As already described, the skin of patients will become increasingly fragile with age. This puts many patients at risk of injury from mechanical stress, from abrasions and skin tears, to more lasting damage caused by more constant pressure, such as pressure ulcers.

The three main causes of mechanical damage are pressure, shearing or friction forces. Often, a combination of all three will be present in patients who develop pressure ulcers.

Patients moving around in bed, when the heels or buttocks are not clear of the bottom sheet, may develop pressure damage.

The degree of mechanical stress experienced by the patient will vary according to loss of muscle bulk, loss of tone, or extreme weight loss which may occur in advanced malignant disease (Swain and Bader, 2002).

Temperature

Wound healing has to take place at the temperature which best supports cell division. The normal body temperature is 37°C, and this is the temperature at which cell division and all cellular activity is optimal. If a wound is exposed, even for short periods, the temperature falls below the required level needed to sustain mitotic activity, slowing down healing. Many wounds occur on peripheral areas and lower limbs. In hypothermic patients, there is a risk of slow wound progress due, in part, to temperature, but also to decreased peripheral circulation. Temperature should be considered when assessing wound progress.

Inappropriate use of antimicrobial agents or dressings

The role of antimicrobial products has changed immensely over the past decade and is a subject of ongoing debate. Routine use of antimicrobials should be discouraged to minimise resistance and help prevent hypersensitivity to certain products. Antimicrobials must be used with discretion, based on thorough and accurate wound assessment.

The vast array of antimicrobial wound management products available can make decisions in practice difficult. The question to ask is 'Will the wound benefit from the use of the product?'

Systemic antibiotics should only be used in wounds exhibiting outward signs of infection, or in cases where patients are at risk of systemic infection. Indiscriminate use will again encourage the resistant organisms to emerge.

Modern versions of iodine products and silver are generally considered useful in addressing both established infection and critical colonisation of wounds.

Radiotherapy

Radiation therapy is used to directly infiltrate tumour and/or tumour deposits and halt the growth of the malignancy. Despite the accuracy of the therapy, there is often an area of the skin which is effectively burned by the radiation. Normal cell reproduction is also affected by the treatment as it is non-selective and, therefore, wound healing is often difficult following courses of the therapy.

The damage may involve capillaries and basal cells and lead to local skin reactions (Sitton, 1992).

Radiation therapy also inhibits epithelial tissue and can generate erythema. It is often painful for the patient

Conclusion

This chapter illustrates a number of significant risk factors that can contribute to delayed wound healing. Diabetes mellitus, poor nutrition, renal disease and the use of steroids need to be understood, not just as individual risk factors, but as part of a composite risk. Patients who suffer from one or other chronic illness may live in disadvantaged social circumstances. Elderly patients may have multiple chronic illnesses and, moreover, be poorly-motivated or equipped to sustain self-care. Wounds heal more slowly (or not at all) where risk factors accumulate. If nurses are to assess wound healing risk factors in a coherent way, it is important to think beyond the wound site.

Using a zone approach to the assessment of risk represents a first step in wound healing risk management. While the approach does not quantify the risks, or calculate the ways in which multiple risks accentuate the challenge to wound care, it does alert nurses to the need to think practically as well as holistically. There will be times when the weight of accumulating risk factors recommends early referral to specialist wound care facilities. Or, it may prompt us to work in several different ways to enhance the chances of successful wound healing. Thinking laterally, the protein we provide to patients, the lighting we improve in their homes, or the blood sugar levels that help to control the person with diabetes, may be every bit as influential as the wound dressing we recommend.

References

Adam K, Oswald I (1983) Protein synthesis, bodily renewal and the sleep-wake cycle. *Clinical Science* **65**(6): 561–7

Alinovi A, Bassissi P, Pini M (1986) Systemic administration of antibiotics in the management of venous ulcers. *J Am Acad Dermatol* **15**: 186–91

Browne A, Dow G, Sibbald RG (2001) Cutaneous wound repair. In: Falanga V, ed. *Infected Wounds*. Martin Dunitz, London: 213–5

Byrne J (1999) Rheumatology part 2: the role of medication. *Prof Nurse* **14**(5): 355–8

Cullen B, Smith R, McCulloch E *et al* (2002) Mechanism of action of Promogran, a protease modulating matrix for the treatment of diabetic foot ulcers. *Wound Rep Regen* **10**(1): 16–25

Cutting KF (1994) Factors affecting wound healing. *Nurs Standard* **8**(50): 33–6

Cutting KF, Harding KG (1994) Criteria for identifying wound infection. *J Wound Care* **3**(4): 198–201

Cutting KF (1998) The identification of infection in granulating wounds by registered nurses. *J Clin Nurs* **7**: 539–46

Cutting KF (2001) A dedicated follower of fashion? Topical medications and wounds. *Br J Nurs* **10**(15) Silver Supplement: 9–16

Cutting KF, White R (2002) Maceration of the skin: 1; The nature and causes of skin maceration. *J Wound Care* **11**(7): 275–8

Dow G, Browne A, Sibbald RG (1999) Infection in chronic wounds: controversies in diagnosis and treatment. *Ostomy Wound Management* **45**(8): 23–7, 29–40

Dyson M *et al* (1988) Comparison of the effects of moist and dry conditions on dermal repair. *J Invest Derm* **91**: 729–33

Falanga V (1999) Overview of chronic wounds and recent advances. *Dermatol Therapeutics* **9**: 7–17

Fernie GR, Dornan J (1976) The problems of clinical trials with new systems for preventing or healing decubetis. In: Kenedi RM *et al*, eds. *Bedsore Bioechanics*. Macmillan, London: 315–20

Gardner SE, Frantz RA, Doebbeling BN (2001) The validity of the clinical signs and symptoms used to identify localized chronic wound infection. *Wound Rep Regen* **9**(3): 178–86

Gilchrist B (1999) Wound infection. In: Miller M, Glover D, eds. *Wound Management, Theory and Practice*. Nursing Times Books, London: 96–106

Glaser R, Kiecolt-Glaser JK, Marucha PT *et al* (1999) Stress-related changes in pro-inflammatory cytokine production in wounds. *Arch Gen Psych* **56**(5): 450–6

Gray D, Cooper P (2001) Nutrition and wound healing: what is the link? *J Wound Care* **10**(3): 86–9

Hart J, Silcock D, Gunnigle J *et al* (2002) The role of oxidised regenerated cellulose/collagen in wound repair. Effects in vitro on fibroblast biology and effects in vivo on a model of compromised wound healing. *Int Biochem Cell Biol* **34**(12): 1557–70

Hinman CD, Maibach H (1963) Effect of air exposure and occlusion on experimental human skin wounds. *Nature* **200**: 377–9

Holden-Lund C (1988) Effects of relaxation with guided imagery on surgical stress and wound healing. *Res Nurs Health* **11**: 235–44

Huovinen S, Kotilainen P, Jarvinen H *et al* (1994) Comparison of ciprofloxicin or trimethoprin therapy for venous leg ulcers; results of a pilot study. *J Am Acad Dermatol* **31**: 279–81

Hunt TK (1969) The effect of vitamin A on reversing the inhibitory effects of cortisone in the healing of open wounds. *Am J Surg* **170**: 633–41

Jacobson RG, Flowers FP (1996) Skin changes with ageing and disease. *Wound Rep Regen* **4**(3): 311–15

Jensen JA, Goodson WH, Williams H, Hunt TK (1991) Cigarette smoking decreases tissue oxygen. *Arch Surg* **126**: 1131–4

Jacobson RG, Flowers FP. 1996. Skin changes with aging and disease. *Wound Rep Regen* **4**(3): 311–5

Jorgensen LN, Kallehave F Christensen E, Siana JE Gottrup F (1998) Less collagen production in smokers. *Surgery* **123**: 450–5

Kane DP, Krasner D (1997) Wound healing and wound management. In: Krasner D, Kane D, eds. *Chronic Wound Care*, 2nd edn. Wayne PA, Health Management Publications, Inc

Kanzler MH, Gorsulowsky DC, Swanson NA (1986) Basic mechanisms in the healing cutaneous wound. *J Dermatologic Surg Oncol* **12**: 1156–64

Kiecolt-Glaser J, Marucha PT, Malarkey W, Mercado A, Glaser R (1995) Slowing of wound healing by psychological stress. *Lancet* **346**: 1194–6

Kindlen S, Morison M (1997) The physiology of wound healing. In: Morison M, Moffatt C, Bridel-Nixon J, Bale S, eds. *Nursing Management of Chronic Wounds*. Mosby, London

Kinsella K (1996) Demographic aspects. In: Ebrahim S, Kalache A, eds. *Epidemiology in Old Age*. British Medical Journal/World Health Organisation Publication, London

Kozol RA, Fromm D, Ackerman NB, Chung R (1986) Wound closure in obese patients. *Surg Gynecol Obstet* **162**(5): 442–4

Kyriazis M (1994) Age and reason: theory of ageing and ageing mechanisms. *Nurs Times* **90**(18): 60–2

Larsen K, Fabrin J, Holstein PE (2001) Incidence and management of ulcers in diabetic Charcot feet. *J Wound Care* **10**(8): 323–8

Lennard-Jones JE (1992) *A positive approach to nutrition as treatment, report of a working party on the role of enteral and parenteral feeding in hospital and home.* King's Fund, London

Lotti T, Rodofill C, Benci M, Menchin G (1998) Wound healing problems associated with cancers. *J Wound Care* **7**(2): 81–4

Mani R, Falanga V, Shearman CP, Sandeman D (1999) *Clinical Aspects of Lower Limb Ulceration in Chronic Wound Healing*. WB Saunders, London

Martin MTM (1998) Sub-clinical malnutrition and its possible association with the rate of wound healing in people aged 60 years and over. In: Leaper D, ed. Proceedings of the 7th European Conference in Wound Management. EMAP Healthcare Ltd, London: 129–33

Mendez-Eastman S (1998) Negative pressure wound therapy. *Plastic Surg Nurs* **1**: 27–9, 33–7

Moore K (2003) Compromised wound healing. *Br J Community Nurs* **8**(6): 1–4

Miller M, Dyson M (1996) *Understanding Wound Healing*. Professional Nurse Publications, EMAP Healthcare, London: 62–4

Newton D, Leese G, Harrison D, Belch J (2001) Microvascular abnormalities in diabetic foot ulcers. *Diabetic Foot* **4**(3): 141–6

Office of Populaton Censuses and Surveys (1996) *Living in Britain: results for the 1994 General Household Survey*. HMSO, London

Olde Damink SWM, Soeters PB (1997) Nutrition and wound healing. *Nurs Times* **93**(30): suppl 1–6

O'Meara SO, Cullum N, Majid M, Sheldon T (2001) Systematic review of antimicrobial agents used for chronic wounds. *Br J Surg* **88**: 4–21

Parks WC (1999) Matrix metalloproteinases in repair. *Wound Rep Regen* **7**: 423–33

Perkins P (1992) Wound dehiscence: cause and care. *Nurs Standard* **6**(34): 12–4

Pinchcofski–Devin G, Kaminski MV (1986) Correlation of pressure sores and nutritional status. *J Am Geriatr Soc* **34**: 435–40

Plewa MC (1990) Altered host response and special infections in the elderly. *Emerg Med Clin North Am* **8**(2): 193–206

Sibbald RG, Williams D, Orsted HL *et al* (2000) Preparing the wound bed, debridement, bacterial balance and moisture balance. *Ostomy Wound Management* **46**(11): 14–35

Sitton–Kent L, Gilchrist B (1993) The intake of nutrients by hospitalised pensioners with chronic wounds. *J Adv Nurs* **18**(12): 1962–7

Sorensen LT, Neilsen HB, Kharazmi A, Karlsmark T, Gottrup F (2003) Abstinence from smoking enhances neutrophil bactericidal activity and reduces wound infection. EWMA Conference, Pisa, Italy

Swain ID, Bader DL (2002) The measurement of interface pressure and its role in soft tissue breakdown. *J Tissue Viability* **12**(4): 132–44

Springhouse Corporation (1998) *Handbook of Medical Surgical Nursing*, 2nd edn. PA Springhouse Corporation, New York

Thomas S (1992) *Current Practices in the Management of Fungating Lesions and Radiation Damaged Skin*. The Surgical Materials Testing Laboratory, Brigend

Thomas D (2000) Matrix metalloproteinases, tissue inhibitors of metalloproteinases and wound bed status. In: Cherry G, Harding K, Ryan initial, eds. *Wound Bed Preparation, International congress and symposium series.* Royal Society of Medicine Press, London: 17–21

Timmons JP (2003) Factors that delay wound healing. *Primary Health Care J* **13**(5): 434–9

Walsh M (2001) Caring for the patient with a disorder of the renal system. In: Walsh M, ed. *Clinical Nursing and Related Science.* 6th edn. Ballière Tindall, Edinburgh: 612–3

White R (2003) An historical overview of the use of silver in wound management. In: White R, ed. *The Silver Book.* Quay Books, MA Healthcare, London

Winter G (1962) Formation of the scab and rate of epithelialisation in the skin of the young domestic pig. *Nature* **193**: 293–5

Self-assessment exercises

Look back to *Figure 3.1* (p. 48) and think about a patient with a wound that you have recently nursed. Reproduce the three concentric circles of the zonal diagram and, in the centre one, describe the condition of the wound as you remember it. What progress was being achieved and what were you attempting to achieve in your wound care?

Now consider the systemic zone — physiological and psychological. What were the circumstances here and how did these seem to affect the wound and associated care? For example, did this patient seem able to follow wound care instructions? Lastly, recall the social conditions under which this patient lived and add notes into that ring. What seemed to enhance wound healing and what might have undermined it?

Examine *Figure 3.2* (p. 52), what do you see? What would you try to observe about the circulation to this woman's leg, the condition of her skin more generally, and the room in which she sits. Was it well lit, clean and warm?

You are caring for a patient who has a wound and suffers from venous disease, chronic obstructive pulmonary disease and arthritis (*Figure 3.2*). What points would you wish to discuss with the patient's doctor? What would you explain about the wound in order to arrive at the artful compromise in patient treatment and care?

Chapter 4

Applied Wound Management

David Gray, Richard White, Pam Cooper, Andrew Kingsley

Introduction

Assessing a patient with a wound involves accurate assessment of both the wound and the patient's health status. Failure to carry out such assessment, or to ensure that the treatments are relevant to the individual, could cause delayed wound healing or serious complications for the patient. This chapter poses seven questions to guide the practitioner through the assessment of a patient with a wound. To assess the wound, the concept of Applied Wound Management is utilised.

Patient assessment

1. What kind of wound am I looking at?

It is impossible to treat a wound appropriately if the practitioner is unable to identify the structures visible in the wound, and understand the factors which prevent wound healing. Identifying the type of tissue present, and the implications of that tissue on healing are key skills. Wounds, such as pressure ulcers or diabetic foot ulcers may occur in similar locations and present in a similar manner, but they require different management. Failing to identify the type of wound correctly can cause complications, which may be life-threatening. By utilising the Applied Wound Management System, a systematic assessment of the wound can be conducted and treatment objectives identified.

2. Why has this wound developed?

Wounds develop as a result of specific circumstances. For example, a wound could be from some form of trauma in the case of pressure ulcers, or because of an underlying medical condition, such as venous hypertension in venous leg ulceration. Failing to identify and deal with the cause is likely to lead to deterioration in the wound and delay healing. Alternatively, the wound may be a symptom of a disease or condition which requires urgent medical attention or surgery.

3. What else is happening to this person?

Wound healing cannot be achieved without considering the patient's overall health. Conditions such as cardiac failure, diabetes and other chronic conditions can have a major impact on healing. It is also recognised that the individual's psychosocial circumstances can significantly effect the healing process. The practitioner may fail to identify barriers to healing if he/she treats the wound in isolation, without reference to the patient's physical or mental health and social circumstances.

4. What are the potential outcomes for the person with this wound?

While wound healing is the expected outcome for most patients, this is not always possible or desirable. In situations where there is insufficient blood supply to the wound, as in the case of peripheral vascular disease (PVD), it may be impossible to achieve healing and, to attempt to do so would be detrimental to the patient. Wounds associated with malignancy are likely to require symptom management. It is important to establish at an early stage the outcome that is appropriate for the patient.

5. What is the best management for this person?

The best management plan will become apparent as an understanding of the patient's circumstances is reached and a thorough assessment of the wound is conducted. This is likely to involve far more than the selection of a wound dressing, but may require further investigation, referral to a specialist service, or a combination of treatments, such as specific wound management products together with compression bandaging and lifestyle changes.

6. Do I have the skills to manage this person's wound?

In some situations, the wound may have developed as a result of a medical condition and require a specialist referral. Alternatively, surgery may be indicated, or specialist investigations or treatments which are beyond the ability or scope of the practitioner. It is an essential element of professional practice that the practitioner reflects on his/her own ability and knowledge, and recognises his/her limitations. This ensures that the practitioner works within their professional competence, and that the patient with a wound is assured of the best management.

7. How will I monitor the progress of this wound?

A standardised method of evaluation facilitates accurate assessment of the wound, as it provides a baseline against which progress can be measured. Precise, detailed documentation, including wound dimensions in centimetres, form the basis of professional practice in wound management. The practitioner should be alert to any changes in the health status of the individual, as well as the wound, so that a specialist referral can be made if required

Wound assessment

The Applied Wound Management (AWM) framework utilises three different continuums, each relating to a key wound parameter:

❖ **Wound Healing Continuum (WHC):** is represented by the tissues in the wound and is a colour-based continuum.

❖ **Wound Infection Continuum (WIC):** is subdivided into named stages representing varying host responses to bioburden, each identified by clinical cues.

❖ **Wound Exudate Continuum (WEC):** is represented by volume and consistency parameters, and each can be graded according to a 'matrix' continuum.

This practical application to everyday wound care enables the practitioner to approach wound assessment logically and systematically. Increased workloads across the NHS require decision-making to be systematic, clear and coherent. The AWM system aids this type of decision-making, reducing the risk of poor practice and litigation.

Using the Wound Healing Continuum to assess tissue

Wound tissue types

If left to heal by secondary intention, the tissues in a wound (within the wound bed and margins) indicate the relevant pathologies present, reflect the state of healing and, consequently, the success of the management approach. Thus, a black wound (as opposed to black skin changes in melanoma, gangrene or frostbite) indicates the presence of eschar or necrosis (Bale, 1997). Wound eschar is full-thickness, dry, devitalised (dead) tissue that has arisen through prolonged local ischaemia. In relation to pressure ulcers, eschar might arise after a sudden large vessel occlusion caused by shearing injury (Witkowski and Parish, 1982). Unless removed, the eschar will delay healing, as healing cannot proceed effectively without a moist wound environment (Winter, 1962; Parnham, 2002).

Yellow and fibrous wound tissue that adheres to the wound bed and cannot be removed on irrigation is known as slough (Tong, 1999). This adherent, fibrous material is derived from the proteins, fibrin and fibrinogen (Tong, 1999). In combination with wound exudate, it serves as an ideal environment for bacterial growth and, consequently, infection (Colebrook _et al_, 1960; O'Brien, 2002; Davies, 2004). It also impairs healing by restricting re-epithelialisation (Kubo _et al_, 2001). The clinical objective of managing a sloughy wound is to debride (Tong, 1999; Hampton, 2005).

The red, moist tissue in a wound is a combination of new blood vessel growth (angiogenesis), and a matrix of fibroblasts (connective tissue or dermal cells), known as granulation tissue. This is usually indicative of a healing wound and is often accompanied by signs of re-epithelialisation (epidermal regrowth) (Gray _et al_, 2003). It is important to remember that not all red wounds are healthy; they may be critically colonised and non-healing/static, or show evidence of haemolytic bacteria (if a dull brick-red colour) (Dowsett _et al_, 2004).

The approach taken in the Wound Healing Continuum is to incorporate intermediate colour combinations between the four key colours (_Figure 4.1_). To use this system to the optimum clinical benefit, it is first important to identify the colour that is furthest to the left of the continuum. For example, if the wound contains yellow slough and red granulation tissue, it would be defined as a 'yellow/red wound'. A key objective of the consequent wound management plan would be to remove the yellow tissue and promote the growth of red granulation tissue (Gray _et al_, 2005). In this instance, the management plan should focus on removal of the yellow sloughy tissue, and promotion of the red granulation tissue. As this objective is achieved, the wound can progress along the continuum towards the right, to the 'pink/healing' status. It is important to remember that, in addition to this focus on the wound bed and margins, care must be taken to protect the skin surrounding the wound. The interaction of otherwise healthy skin with exudate can lead to maceration and wound enlargement (White and Cutting, 2003).

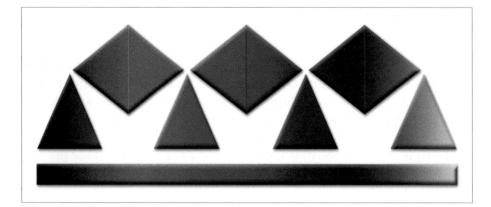

Figure 4.1: The Wound Healing Continuum

Identifying and obtaining treatment objectives

Debridement

Where the wound exhibits dead tissue, eg. black, black/yellow, yellow, or yellow/red, a key treatment aim should be the debridement of the devitalised tissue, unless contraindicated by the patient's overall physical condition or disease process, such as PVD (European Tissue Repair Society [ETRS], 2003). There are debridement options available to the practitioner and each patient requires individual management. Many different clinical presentations and challenges are likely to face the practitioner when a wound needs to be debrided, for example, the volume and viscosity of exudate present, or the presence of infection, must be considered. The types of treatment available can be divided into three separate categories:

- active
- autolytic (moisture donation).
- autolytic (moisture absorption).

Active debridement

❖ **Surgical debridement:** This involves removing the dead tissue from the wound bed. It is usually carried out under surgical conditions in locations such as operating theatres, and results in a bleeding wound bed. This form of debridement is carried out by surgeons/ podiatrists and specialist nurses, using surgical instruments such as scalpels and forceps. It removes dead tissue and results in an inflammatory response from the wound, thus stimulating healing (Bale, 1997).

❖ **Sharp debridement:** This is the removal of dead tissue. This technique involves debulking the wound of slough and necrotic tissue (ie. reducing the amount of dead tissue within the wound). As the objective is not to create a bleeding wound bed (that is, the complete removal of dead tissue), some slough and necrosis are left. The removal of dead tissue, as may be achieved by sharp debridement, is essential for wound healing (O'Brien, 2002). This process, unlike surgical debridement, is usually carried out at the patient's bedside, or in the patient's own home. It requires the use of surgical instruments, such as a specialist wound debridement pack.

❖ **Larval therapy:** The use of maggot larvae to debride the wound of dead tissue has become a mainstream therapy in the UK during the past decade. The larvae liquefy the dead tissue and, where the treatment is successful, can result in rapid debridement (Thomas _et al_, 1998).

Autolytic debridement

Autolytic debridement is the removal of devitalised tissue from the wound by means of the body's own enzymes operating in a moist environment. Where tissue can be kept moist it will naturally degrade and deslough from the underlying healthy structures. This process is facilitated by enzymes (matrix metalloproteinases) which disrupt the proteins that bind the dead tissue to the body (Schultz _et al_, 2003). The process can be enhanced by the application of wound management products which promote a moist environment. These products can be divided into two categories: those that donate moisture to the dead tissue, and those that absorb excess moisture produced by the body. Both are designed to facilitate the autolytic debridement process.

❖ **Autolytic (moisture donation):** The group of products listed in *Figure 4.2* facilitate autolytic debridement by donating moisture to the dead tissue, and are designed to facilitate the natural process of autolysis. Hydrocolloids, hydrogels, honey and silver sulfadiazine cream donate moisture to the wound and thus enhance the process of debridement (Cooper *et al*, 2003). These products can be used at all stages of the Wound Healing Continuum, and some also have antimicrobial activity. The use of antimicrobial products should always be based on clinical need and not as a matter of routine.

❖ **Autolytic (moisture absorption):** The groups of products listed in *Figure 4.2* (alginates, cadexomer iodine and Hydrofiber®, ConvaTec) facilitate autolytic debridement by absorbing moisture from the wound (exudate), while ensuring that the necrotic tissue does not dry out (Cooper *et al*, 2003). By absorbing excess exudate, these products avoid damage from maceration to the surrounding skin. As with the moisture-donating products, some of the products within the moisture-absorption group also have an antimicrobial effect. *Figure 4.2* indicates where these products can be used across the Wound Healing Continuum.

Treatment Options		Black	Black/Yellow	Yellow	Yellow/Red	Red	Red/Pink	Pink
Active								
	Surgical debridement							
	Sharp debridement							
	Larval therapy							
Autolytic (moisture donation)								
	Hydrocolloids							
	Hydrogels							
	Honey #							
	Silver sulfadiazine #							
Autolytic (moisture absorption)								
	Alginates *							
	Cadexomer iodine #							
	Hydrofiber® *							

Figure 4.2: Wound management treatments: debridement
These products have an antimicrobial effect
* Some products in this category have antimicrobial effects

Clinical use of debridement techniques

Treatments from more than one group (_Figure 4.2_) may be required to achieve full debridement of the wound. The heel pressure ulcer presented in _Figure 4.3_ shows necrotic tissue which has been rehydrated using an autolytic (moisture-donating) treatment. This results in necrotic eschar lifting at the wound margins and separating from the slough below. The necrotic tissue is categorised as 'black' on the Wound Healing Continuum.

In _Figure 4.4_, the wound has been subjected to sharp debridement and the necrotic tissue removed to leave the slough below exposed. The wound is now categorised as a 'yellow' wound on the Wound Healing Continuum. No bleeding or pain has been caused. Following sharp debridement, the patient is treated with a moisture-donating product (eg. hydrogel) to continue the process of autolytic debridement.

The wound in _Figure 4.5_ is producing high levels of moisture which need to be absorbed. The wound bed is covered with slough which requires debriding. The wound is categorised as a 'yellow/red' wound on the Wound Healing Continuum. By utilising an autolytic (moisture-absorption) treatment, the wound is successfully debrided and has moved on to the next stage of the Healing Continuum — 'red' (_Figure 4.6_).

Granulation and epithelialisation

Where a wound has been categorised as 'red' or 'red/pink', the main objective is the promotion of granulation tissue and then epithelialisation. Granulation (red) and epithelial (pink) tissue are the final two stages of the Wound Healing Continuum. Granulation tissue is formed in the wound bed as a result of the action of fibroblasts stimulated by the growth factors provided by macrophages. Angiogenesis, the development of new capillary buds, leads to the development of new blood vessels. Granulation presents as a red, uneven surface. It is highly vascular and needs to be kept moist to facilitate its growth. As granulation develops in the wound, the margins begin to show signs of epithelial growth and pink tissue forms across the surface of the granulation tissue. This is the final stage of healing. This layer is only one cell thick and requires protection from desiccation and trauma.

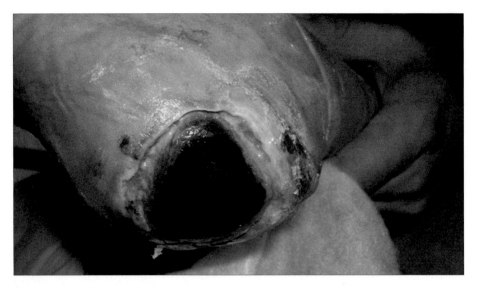

Figure 4.3: Black wound

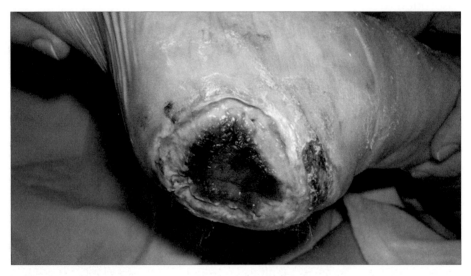

Figure 4.4: Black/yellow wound post sharp debridement

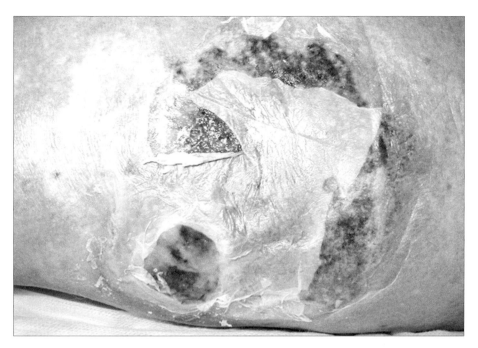

Figure 4.5: Yellow/red wound

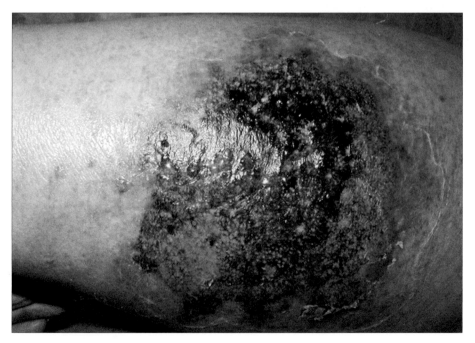

Figure 4.6: Red wound

Both granulation and epithelial tissue need to be kept moist and protected from trauma. Three different categories of treatment are available when healing by secondary intention: active, moisture donation and moisture absorption. Many products can either donate or absorb moisture in a granulating wound and, for the purposes of this chapter, they have been categorised in relation to their main function as interpreted by the authors. Some active treatments, such as skin grafting and skin substitutes, have not been included in this chapter.

Active treatment

Topical negative pressure therapy (VAC® – vacuum assisted closure) is used in the management of large granulating wounds, particularly cavity wounds. A foam pad is placed into the wound, which is then sealed and negative pressure applied via a vacuum pump. This facilitates the promotion of granulation tissue as well as removing excess exudate (Moore, 2005). As a result of the partial vacuum created by the therapy, exudate is removed from the wound while still maintaining a moist wound environment (Banwell, 1999). Where high exudate levels occur, such as in deep pressure ulcers or dehisced abdominal wounds, VAC® therapy can facilitate exudate management. Angiogenesis can be stimulated by the application of topical negative pressure (Argenta and Morykwas, 1997).

Moisture donation

The fragile nature of granulation tissue means that it has to be kept moist to prevent desiccation and delayed tissue growth. Products such as hydrocolloids, hydrogels and honey, can all deliver moisture to the wound bed, thus supporting granulation. Hydrocolloids, sheet hydrogels and sheet honey dressings can also provide an element of moisture absorption (Cooper, *et al*, 2003), but this is not their main function which is that of moisture donation. Some of these products may also have an antimicrobial action.

Moisture absorption

An excess of moisture on the wound bed can lead to maceration of the wound margins and delayed healing (Cameron and Powell, 1992). The products listed in *Figure 4.7* (alginates, cadexomer iodine, collagen products, foams and Hydrofiber®) absorb exudate, providing the ideal environment for the promotion of granulation tissue and epithelialisation of the wound. Some of the products may have an antimicrobial capability.

Treatment Options			Black/Yellow	Yellow	Yellow/Red	Red	Red/Pink	Pink
Active	Topical negative pressure							
Autolytic (moisture donation)								
	Hydrocolloids							
	Hydrogels							
	Honey #							
Autolytic (moisture absorption)								
	Alginates *							
	Cadexomer iodine #							
	Collagen products*							
	Foam*							
	Hydrofiber® *							

Figure 4.7: Wound management treatments: granulation and epithelialisation
\# These products have an antimicrobial effect
* Some products in this category have antimicrobial effects

Promotion of granulation and epithelial tissue in clinical practice

In *Figure 4.8*, the patient has presented with an abrasion to the knee. The wound is categorised as 'red' on the Wound Healing Continuum. An accurate assessment of the patient would reveal whether or not the wound is producing sufficient exudate to facilitate healing. Depending on the outcome of the assessment, the correct product selection will lead to a 'pink' wound as seen in *Figure 4.9*.

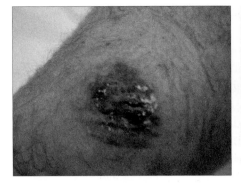

Figure 4.8: Red wound

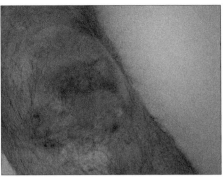

Figure 4.9: Pink wound

Conclusion

The Wound Healing Continuum supports a systematic assessment of the wound, and the identification of clear treatment objectives. Where there is dead tissue, debridement is likely to be the treatment objective unless otherwise contraindicated by the patient's condition. Where debridement is identified as the treatment objective, the clinical judgement of the practitioner is needed to decide the method of debridement required. As stated, it is likely that more than one method will be used as the wound progresses to a 'red' wound bed. It is important that treatments are prescribed only after a holistic assessment of the patient's needs has been carried out.

Similarly, following a systematic assessment of wounds in the 'yellow/red' to 'pink' categories, the treatments must be selected to promote granulation and meet the needs of the patient. Ensuring the rapid growth of granulation and epithelial tissue, not only reduces the time required to achieve healing, but also reduces the risk of wound infection (Gray et al, 2003). A balanced, moist environment can be achieved using many different treatments; however, it is vital that the selection of such treatments is underpinned by regular, accurate assessments.

Using the Wound Infection Continuum to assess bioburden

While all chronic wounds left to heal by secondary intention will contain bacteria throughout, it is the delicate balance between the host (immune) response and the pathogen that must be managed if infection is to be avoided (Casadevall and Pirofski, 2000). The mere presence of colonising bacteria in a chronic wound is usually of no clinical significance, as this level of bioburden does not impair healing (Leaper, 1994).

From a clinical management perspective, it is the recognition of the state of the wound — with respect to the infection status — that is the challenge. Research informs us of the bacteria that contribute to the wound bioburden, and of the criteria for infection. However, the key to good wound management is to avoid infection. It is important to recognise the subtle signs and symptoms that precede infection, and to intervene accordingly. These factors are included in the evolving 'Wound Infection Continuum' and the related treatment guidelines.

Wounds that do not exhibit the classical signs of infection may become indolent through the effects of bioburden and, although they might benefit from an antimicrobial strategy, either topical or systemic, they often go untreated. Improving the clinician's ability to make a clinical diagnosis requires a consolidation of microbiological status and the incorporation of clinical signs and symptoms into an easily understood package. It could be argued that there is no clear consensus as to what constitutes the clinical signs of wound infection; however, these have recently been clarified (Cutting and White, 2005; Cutting *et al*, 2005).

Thus, it is necessary to extrapolate the principles of microbiological growth, transmission, and pathological potential developed in the laboratory to the clinical setting. The concept for building a bridge between microbiological theory and clinical practice is called the Wound Infection Continuum. This continuum seeks, in a highly simplified form, to align the states of colonisation, critical colonisation, local infection and spreading infection, with the probable bacterial bioburden and host response, thereby enabling the practitioner to interpret what is happening. In particular, it is possible using the Wound Infection Continuum to guide the appropriate use of the plethora of new antimicrobial therapies that are now available. This makes for good 'prescribing' in terms of both clinical- and cost-effectiveness.

In clinical practice, the main focus is on reducing the high levels of organisms that are causing problems. The ultimate aim is to achieve this without toxicity to healing cells, bacterial resistance, or elevating costs.

The Wound Infection Continuum is a key part of the concept of Applied Wound Management (Gray *et al*, 2005), and represents the varying levels of bioburden in the wound (Kingsley, 2001; White, 2003; Edwards and Harding; 2004). The continuum uses conceptual names for increasingly severe forms of wound bioburden that link with the patient's host (immune) response. The use of the term 'continuum' in this context is not new, and has been used to describe abdominal contamination, infection and sepsis (Schein *et al*, 1997).

Quantification of bioburden may prove difficult, as clinical outcomes rely on the ability of the host to mount an immune response, and this will be different for each individual. Progression along the continuum in the direction of increasing clinical severity denotes increasing bioburden, which only becomes clinically relevant for chronicity once the state of colonisation has been passed. It is crucial to remember that in the wound healing by secondary intention, colonisation is the 'healthy' situation (Edwards and Harding, 2004). Colonised wounds often heal without the need to control bioburden (Leaper, 1994).

The most controversial point on the continuum is that of critical colonisation; a state of delayed healing. This has now been rationalised in a scientific study by Stephens *et al* (2003). Although the authors did not claim this to be the case, their findings strongly suggest that soluble metabolites from anaerobic cocci can give rise to 'delayed healing', through the impaired metabolism of key wound cell populations. Clinical management has been defined as a need for topical, sustained release antimicrobial (not antibiotic) wound dressings (Kingsley, 2003; Bolton and Hermans, 2004).

The quantity and diversity of microbes present in colonisation, critical colonisation and infection are different and dependent upon the degree of the host immune response. Some wounds progress quickly from colonisation to infection via a clinically indistinct 'critical colonisation' state. Other wounds stop at that point and become indolent (Heggers *et al*, 1992; Ennis and Meneses, 2000). Critically colonised wounds will become increasingly 'chronic', or indolent, because cellular cascades are disordered, and there is a biochemical imbalance arising from bacterial metabolism (Wall *et al*, 2002; Stephens *et al*, 2003). Wounds in this state can prove resistant to adjustment with current therapy, as well as to emerging novel therapies such as protease inhibitors, extracellular matrix components and topical growth factors. Thus, early recognition of disordered healing caused commonly, either wholly or partly, by microbes, is vital to achieving good outcomes.

Infection, critical colonisation and colonisation

The Wound Infection Continuum has historically been drawn to show increasing severity of clinical and microbiological states, from left to right (Kingsley, 2001). However, it can be reversed to link with the Wound Healing and Exudate Continuums, so providing a 'global' wound assessment of key presenting features: healing (tissues in the wound); infection (wound bioburden); and, exudate (Gray *et al*, 2005), to promote ease of assessment and documentation of progress in clinical practice. In the original Infection Continuum (Kingsley, 2001), the states of 'sterility' and 'contamination' were included to reflect the presence of microbial growth from the outset of wounding. Sterility represents the absence of any organism in the wound, and is a very unusual situation in wounds healing by secondary intent (Leaper, 1994). For the purpose of clinical practice, understanding this state can be ignored. Similarly, contamination, which means presence of organisms with no active growth and not accompanied by a visible host response, is of no relevance to clinical practice.

The normal microbiological state of a healing wound is that of colonisation, which represents a stable state where growth and death of organisms is balanced or below the immune system's healing disruption threshold (Isenberg, 1998; Heinzelmann *et al*, 2002).

Some authors differentiate infection into 'local' and 'systemic' (Sibbald *et al*, 2000; Edwards and Harding, 2004). This classification has been used to provide guidance on the route of administration for systemic antibiotics. Schultz *et al* (2003) describe four levels of microbial interaction:

- contamination
- colonisation
- critical colonisation
- infection.

Edwards and Harding (2004) include two further levels:

- spreading invasive infection
- septicaemia.

Dow *et al* (1999) and Schultz *et al* (2003) utilise, with other factors, a ring of cellulitis of <2cm to suggest antibiotic treatment via oral route, with extensive cellulitis (by absence of further definition presumed to be >2cm) requiring intravenous therapy.

The use of the word 'systemic' for infection that has spread beyond 2 cm from the wound edge could also be unintentionally misleading. Some wounds have wider zones of peripheral redness, but remain local in character, meaning that the inflammation zone does not continue to extend and the patient does not exhibit systemic infection signs produced by the consequences of bacteraemia, notably fever, rigor, and positive blood culture. Therefore, for the purpose of reconsidering the states to depict on the Wound Infection Continuum, the terms 'local' and 'spreading' infection will be used, denoted by the 2 cm threshold as previously discussed in the literature. Further information on this can be found in *Table 4.1*.

The stages in the Wound Infection Continuum identify different states of microbiological and immunological activity. The change from one state to another depends on many factors (*Table 4.2*).

Each successive stage from left to right on the Continuum (*Figure 4.10*), involves an increase in the quantity of microbes, a new pathogen arrival, an increase in the quantity of virulent organisms, or an increase in the virulence (Wilson *et al*, 2002) of the collective species mixture through bacterial synergy (Bowler *et al*, 2001). The situation may shift in favour of the microorganisms if the host immune response is impaired or suddenly reduced (Bowler, 2002; Heinzelmann *et al*, 2002). In addition, shift may result from the presence of potentiating factors, such as the introduction of foreign bodies that reduce the necessary inoculum needed to produce a worsening microbiological environment.

Abnormal states ←——————→ | ←——→ Healing states ——→

Improving wound ————————————————————→

Table 4.1: Revised Wound Infection Continuum with diagnostic and treatment information

	Spreading infection	Local infection	Critical colonisation	Colonisation
Key local characteristics	>2cm redness with pain (unless insensate).	2cm or less redness with pain. Sudden necrosis on wound bed (red inflammatory zone may not be present).	Static (despite appropriate therapy). No cellulitis.	Expected progression towards healing. No cellulitis (but may be small degree of inflammation in early stages consistent with inflammatory phase – generally not more painful to pressure than background wound pain)
Other local characteristics	Heat. Swelling.	Heat and swelling (can be difficult to identify in small red inflammatory zone).		
Additional local characteristics that may be present in addition to key ones	Extension to main wound at skin level. Blistering (fluid filled). New satellite wounds in red inflammatory zone. Increased wetness. Haemorrhagic patching or spotting in surrounding skin. Purulent exudate*. Maceration, if control of exudate is inadequate. Extensive necrotic and/or sloughing necrotic tissue.	Extension to main wound at skin level. Extension to wound at its base (pocketing). Increased wetness Purulent exudate*. Maceration if control of exudates is inadequate. Extensive necrotic and/or sloughing necrotic tissue. Discolouration of granulation tissue (darkening). Friable bleeding granulation tissue (possibly with very bright red tissue). Foul odour.	Thick slough not responding to standard debridement techniques. Fast returning thick slough after sharp or maggot debridement. Wet wound. Purulent exudates. Maceration if control of exudate is inadequate. Blue/green exudate (*Pseudomonas aeruginosa*). Foul odour. Discolouration of granulation tissue (darkening). Friable bleeding granulation tissue (possibly with very bright red tissue).	Debride damaged tissue under standard therapeutic approaches. Gently moist wound surface. Slough but light and mobile in consistency. Inflammation from initial wounding consistent with expectation for inflammation phase of wound healing, but fading away or gone if wound older. Granulation tissue of healthy red colour. Epithelial tissue with colour different from, but relevant to, normal skin tone. Reducing wound size in last 1–2 weeks.

←———— Abnormal states ————→ ←—|—→ Healing states ———→

Improving wound

———————————————————————————————————→

Table 4.1: continued				
	Spreading infection	Local infection	Critical colonisation	Colonisation
Possible systemic features	Neutrophilia. Rising C-reactive protein. Fever. Rigors. Confusion (in the elderly). Bacteraemia. Tachycardia. Tachypnoea. Lymphangiitis. Lymphadenitis.	Neutrophilia. Rising C-reactive protein.	None.	None.
Suggested treatment	Systemic antibiotics – oral if red zone static and still localised even if > 2 cm – IV if red zone more than an obvious local ring around wound or if actively spreading. Use local formulary. Consider topical antiseptic dressings – at this stage medicated dressings may not be cost- or clinically-effective, though it is clinically reasonable to use them in the diabetic foot ulcer, critically ischaemic wounds, burns, and the severely immuno-compromised patient.	Systemic antibiotics – oral. Use local formulary. Topical antiseptic dressings – normally iodine or silver in formulation, or combination suitable for wet wounds. Locally infected wounds with a necrotic eschar will need a wetter formulation. Adjunctive measures – rapid debridement of necrotic tissue may be necessary, consider relevant strategy, eg. sharp or surgical.	Topical antiseptic dressings – normally iodine or silver in formulation or combination suitable for wet wound. Slow-release formulations are preferred. Medical grade Manuka honey may be considered, especially to control foul odour. Use local formulary. Consider topical antiseptic irrigations – some authors suggest use of dilute vinegar to control *Pseudomonas* if blue/green exudate is present. Adjunctive measures – debridement of necrotic tissue may be necessary. Consider relevant strategy, eg. maggots. Use of anti-protease therapy may be valuable with antimicrobials.	Standard wound therapy and control of underlying aetiological factors (eg. venous hypertension, forces of pressure) as local guidelines. Topical antiseptic dressings – normally, no antimicrobials are necessary, however, prophylaxis may be considered in vulnerable wound groups, such as diabetic foot ulcers or vulnerable immuno-suppressed patients. It can also be considered if the patient has a recurrent history of infection in this wound.

* 'Wound exudate need not be purulent in the setting of infection, as bacterial phospholipases and other enzymes and toxins can rapidly destroy neutrophils, producing the classical watery exudate or "dishwater" pus seen in polymicrobial necrotizing infections'. Dow *et al*, 1999

Table 4.2: Wound treatments and their use across the Wound Infection Continuum					
Mode of action	Product	Spreading infection	Local infection	Critically colonised	Colonised
Active	Alginates with silver				
	Film with silver				
	Cadexomer iodine				
	Hydrocolloids with silver				
	Honey				
	Hydrogel sheets with honey				
	Hydrofiber® with silver				
	Iodine tulle				
	Nanocrystaline silver cloth				
	Silver sulfadiazine cream				
Passive	Activated charcoal cloth				
	Foam with silver				

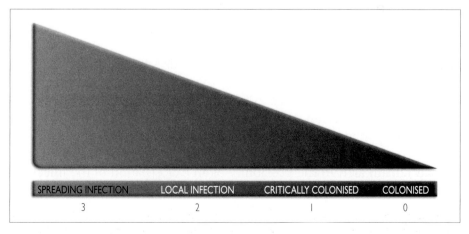

Figure 4.10: The Wound Infection Continuum

Identifying and obtaining treatment objectives

The Wound Infection Continuum is a useful adjunct to the identification of treatment objectives (Gray *et al*, 2005). At different stages of the Continuum, there is likely to be the need for a different treatment objective. It is, however, vital that the identification of such objectives is only arrived at once a full assessment of the patient has taken place, and the implications of the presence of systemic illness or disability understood.

Spreading infection: remove blood stream infection and reduce wound and surrounding tissue bioburden

The presence of a spreading infection associated with an open wound is a systemic disease, which requires a systemic response. As such, the choice of dressing will have little impact on the spreading infection. A systemic response, in the form of antibiotics, is likely to be the treatment of choice, and the wound dressing can seek only to reduce the level of bacteria at the wound surface and thus help prevent re-infection.

Localised infection: remove infection from surrounding tissue and reduce wound bioburden

Where the wound is identified as locally infected, there are a number of options open to the practitioner. Some authors suggest that a localised infection can be treated using topical antimicrobials alone, without recourse to antibiotics (European Pressure Ulcer Advisory Panel [EPUAP], 1999). Others, however, recommend the use of topical antimicrobials with oral antibiotics (Kingsley, 2005). Where the practitioner is satisfied that the patient's overall condition does not suggest a high risk of the infection developing into a spreading infection, it would seem reasonable to adopt a topical antimicrobial-only approach. However, the practitioner should remain alert to the possibility of an exacerbation of the infection, and be prepared to alter the treatment as required. In addition, it would be valuable to set a period of time from the outset in which a reduction of signs and symptoms of infection would be expected to start (eg. <7 days or perhaps by the return of swab culture results), as it would be inappropriate to allow pain to continue unnecessarily or for the wound bed to deteriorate.

Critical colonisation: reduce wound bioburden

In critically colonised wounds, the level of bacteria must be reduced for healing to occur. The topical application of an antimicrobial is probably the most effective way in which to reduce the critically colonised wound bioburden to levels that allow the wound to heal (Cooper, 2004).

Colonised: maintain wound bioburden

Wounds that are identified as colonised do not require any form of topical antimicrobial as the wound bioburden is in a healthy state. Only where there are concerns regarding the patient's immune response, or overall medical condition, should topical antimicrobials be used prophylactically, for example, wounds with a history of recurrent infection, including some diabetic foot ulceration and wounds on lymphoedematous limbs. The indiscriminate prophylactic use of antimicrobials is to be discouraged.

Wound products used to attain treatment objectives

Topical antimicrobial dressings vary in their presentation and action in the wound. As a result, there exists a range of products to aid the practitioner in the control of wound bioburden. The wound treatments available are categorised into two distinct groups: active and passive. These terms describe the mode of the respective dressings, as some dressings donate antimicrobial properties into the wound (active), and others seek to act upon the bacteria as they pass into the dressing (passive). Each form of dressing has its place and it is for practitioners to decide upon the action they require, and the product they select, based on a holistic assessment of the patient.

While the wound dressings available can be divided into two distinct groups by mode of action, there still remain differences in the form such dressings take. In *Table 4.2,* the authors present the dressings in terms of the mode of action, type (eg. Hydrofiber®) and where they may be used across the Wound Infection Continuum. As with any dressing selection, the practitioner must be satisfied that the selection process includes a full assessment of the patient and a full understanding of the dressing's actions.

Conclusion

Accurate assessment of a wound's bioburden and the impact of bacteria on the wound are essential components of wound management. The Wound Infection Continuum encourages practitioners to categorise the level of wound bioburden and identify the relevant treatment objectives. Once these have been identified, it is important that the practitioner is satisfied that treatments selected are suitable for the patient. It is also important to recognise that topical treatments can only be effective when used appropriately, and that their potential to impact on the wound is not misunderstood.

Using the Wound Exudate Continuum to aid wound assessment

Wound healing occurs in four overlapping phases: haemostasis; inflammation; granulation/epithelialisation; and tissue remodelling (Davidson, 1992) (*Chapter 1, pp. 7–9*). Upon injury, vasoconstriction occurs with the aim of reducing blood loss. Haemostasis is achieved by the formation of a clot, which seals the wound. Following haemostasis the inflammatory process begins, during which wound exudate is produced by the tissues surrounding the wound. Normal serous exudate is essential to the healing of the wound (Field and Kerstein, 1994). However, wound exudate is not always 'normal' in terms of volume and/ or consistency; it can present significant management challenges and be a sign of underlying problems relating to the wound bioburden (Cutting, 2004; Cutting and Harding, 1994; Gilchrist, 1999; Vowden and Vowden, 2003, 2004).

Where a wound is healing without complication, exudate can be considered a normal feature. It is produced when blood vessels dilate, post-haemostasis, as part of the inflammatory process. Endothelial cells swell and so open gaps in the vessel wall, permitting extravasation of serous fluid. The presence of this fluid in the tissues surrounding the wound contributes to localised pain, heat, and swelling; symptoms associated with inflammation.

Normal wound exudate is mainly composed of three elements: serous fluid from the leaking blood vessels; debris from local damaged tissue; and growth factors or cytokines (Chen *et al*, 1992; Cutting, 2004; Rogers *et al*, 1995). Wound exudate has a key role to play in the moist wound healing process as it provides not only moisture, but also factors, which effect the removal of dead tissue and the formation of new tissue. Factors such as the underlying condition of the patient, dressing selection, and the pathology of the wound, all affect the production of exudate (White, 2001). Wound exudate has been shown to contain different components at different stages of healing, ie. acute wounds contain growth factors, and chronic wounds contain tissue-degrading enzymes (Cutting, 2004; White, 2001).

Exudate can present significant management challenges. For example, in the case of venous leg ulcers and pressure ulcers, protease enzymes contained in chronic wound exudate (Chen *et al*, 1992) can, if they come into contact with the surrounding skin, result in the development of excoriation and maceration (Cameron and Powell, 1992). Large quantities of exudate can saturate the wound bed (Lamke *et al*, 1997) and peri-wound area causing further maceration (Cutting, 1999; White and Cutting, 2003). Wound exudate can also increase the risk of infection if it soaks through a dressing, thus allowing bacteria to 'strike-through' the wound dressing (this is the passage of exudate from the wound bed through a permeable dressing to appear at the dressing surface – it is believed to be an avenue for bacterial contamination from the environment). However, wound exudate can promote healing if it is managed so as to maintain an optimum moist environment and avoid damage to surrounding skin (Bishop *et al*, 2003).

Exudate will be found at some point in all wounds healing by secondary intention. The volume and viscosity of wound exudate produced by the wound will be influenced by the stage of healing, and the presence or absence of factors such as infection. Wounds healing without complication by secondary intention will gradually reduce their production of exudate as the healing process progresses.

Assessing exudate

Traditionally, exudate has been described in terms of its perceived volume, eg. as light/low, moderate, or heavy (Watret, 1997). This form of assessment is subjective and difficult to quantify in the absence of significant investigation, such as the weighing of dressings pre- and post-use (Thomas, 1997). Vowden and Vowden (2003, 2004) suggest that exudate volume should not be viewed in isolation, but in conjunction with viscosity. By considering both these aspects, an insight can be gained into the underlying condition of the wound and of the patient. They are indicative of the infection status (Cutting, 2004).

The authors suggest that wound exudate volume and viscosity be assessed by:

- considering the exudate that is retained within the dressing
- noting the number of dressing changes required in forty-eight hours
- visual inspection of the wound.

This approach to assessment is complementary to current management strategies, such as the six 'Cs' proposed by Vowden and Vowden (2003) (*Table 4.3*).

Table 4.3: Exudate management strategy based on the six 'Cs', adapted from Vowden and Vowden, 2004					
Cause	Control	Components	Containment	Correction	Complications
Systemic	Whether effective	Bacterial	Dressing seal. At the wound	Bioburden control	Skin protection
Local	systemic or local control	Necrotic	surface, with the dressing	Debride-	Protein loss
Wound-related	possible	Chemical composition	and away from the wound	ment	Pain
		Volume and viscosity			Odour
		pH			

The Wound Exudate Continuum (*Figure 4.11*) is offered as an aid to quantifying the volume and viscosity of wound exudate. The gradings for both of these features are 'high', 'medium' and 'low', and allow wound exudate to be categorised by a numerical score. For example, a wound with exudate of low volume and of medium viscosity would be in the low/medium category and would score 4 (placing it in the low exudate [green] portion of the continuum). Any score in the green zone should be seen as advantageous to wound healing.

If the wound exudate score is 6, then this places the wound in the amber zone. Wounds that are assessed as being in the amber zone require careful consideration, as this category could either indicate an improvement or deterioration in the wound's condition. For example, if the previous recording had been in the green zone, the practitioner should seek to identify why the wound has moved (deteriorated) into the amber zone. A change in score to red from amber, ie. a deterioration, may be because of an alteration in the wound bioburden, indicating critical colonisation or the development of an infection. However, if the previous score had been in the red zone, an amber score would indicate an improvement in the condition of the wound. Any score in the red zone should be investigated urgently as this may indicate local or spreading infection, particularly if the previous score had not been in this zone.

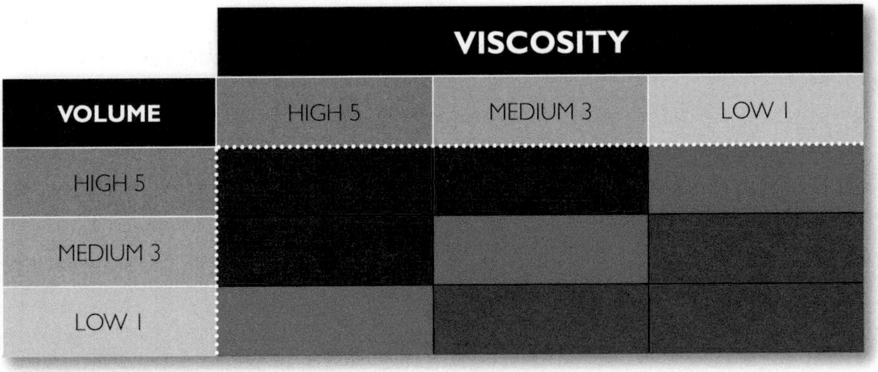

VOLUME	VISCOSITY		
	HIGH 5	MEDIUM 3	LOW 1
HIGH 5			
MEDIUM 3			
LOW 1			

Figure 4.11: The Wound Exudate Continuum

Identifying and obtaining treatment objectives

When reviewing the wound, the exudate on the dressing and present in the wound should be assessed using the questions outlined in *Table 4.4*. This is a highly subjective assessment and should be used to guide clinical judgement and not replace it. Any wound assessed as having both high viscosity and high volume of wound exudate, would score a full ten points and be regarded as causing serious concern. It is likely that such a wound may indicate a spreading infection, sinus or fistula formation, or some other cause for concern. The overriding aim of the wound exudate continuum is to encourage a systematic approach to wound care and to support clinical decision-making. Regardless of the zone, the assessment points to the treatment objectives will fall into one of three categories:

1. Absorb moisture.
2. Maintain current moisture balance.
3. Donate moisture.

When these objectives are added to the objectives identified using the Wound Healing and Wound Infection Continuums, a clear picture of the overall treatment objectives is achieved.

Table 4.4: Exudate assessment: questions to ask	
Questions	Answers
How often has the dressing been changed over the past 48 hours?	Provides an indication as to the volume of exudate being produced
Has there been any leakage from the dressing?	This may provide information on the suitability of the dressing used, and give an indication of the volumes of exudate being produced
Is there any residue on the surface of the wound dressing?	High viscosity exudate is likely to be found on the surface of a wound dressing
Have the margins become macerated?	Maceration is usually associated with high volumes of exudate, and/or prolonged wear time
Is there any exudate on the wound bed?	High viscosity exudate is more likely to be found adhering to the wound bed
Can the staff or patient offer any information regarding the nature of exudate observed over 48 hours?	Often an asssessment is difficult because dressings have been removed or the patient bathed before an assessment

Once an assessment has been carried out and a colour zone identified using the Wound Exudate Continuum, it is possible to identify which product may be suitable using *Figure 4.12*. In *Figure 4.12*, the products have been categorised according to their primary function. Products with an antimicrobial function have been identified by an asterisk. These may be particularly useful where infection or critical colonisation is thought to be present.

Function	Product	Red	Amber	Green
Devices/dressings				
	Topical negative pressure (VAC®)			
	Wound Manager™			
Primary dressings				
	Alginates *			
	Capillary			
	Hydrofiber®*			
Primary/secondary dressings				
	Foams*			
	Films*			
	Hydrocolloids* #			
	Hydrofiber®*			
	Hydrogels* #			

Figure 4.12: Exudate management options
* Denotes where some of the products within this category contain an antimicrobial function
# Denotes products which can donate moisture to the wound where there is insufficient moisture

Product functions

Devices/dressings

In *Figure 4.12*, the first category of products are those which can be described as devices/dressings. In this category there are two different products. First, VAC® (topical negative pressure), which works by applying negative pressure to a wound bed and thus removing the exudate via a tube to a canister. This product can function across the spectrum of exudate zones. A Wound Manager™ (ConvaTec) is a device similar in construction to a colostomy bag, which acts as a reservoir where there are large amounts of exudate. Generally, the Wound Manager™ has a short-term application in acute situations such as dehisced abdominal wounds.

Primary dressings

These dressings are applied directly to the wound bed and absorb exudate. Two classes of dressings have an antimicrobial function when combined with silver; namely, silver alginate and Hydrofiber® plus silver. The capillary dressing has no antimicrobial function, but has a large capacity to absorb fluid and wick it away from the wound bed. All of these primary dressings require a secondary dressing to cover them.

Primary/secondary dressings

The dressings in these categories can be applied as primary dressings (which do not require a secondary dressing), such as the hydrocolloids, hydrogel sheets or film dressings. Foam dressings can act as a primary dressing, but are also frequently used as secondary dressings, absorbing exudate which has passed through the primary dressing. Some products in these categories contain antimicrobial agents, and there are products which can also donate moisture to the wound bed as required.

Conclusion

The Wound Exudate Continuum provides the user with a systematic approach to wound exudate, going beyond simply guessing the volume of exudate produced. The nature of wound exudate gives an indication of the health of the wound and assists in the identification of different levels of bioburden. The Wound Exudate Continuum provides a framework for the practitioner to accurately assess the situation. It can also facilitate the identification of clear treatment objectives which, when used with the other components of Applied Wound Management, provides a systematic approach to wound management.

The values attached to the different levels of exudate are designed to provide the practitioner with an aid to assessment, and not to replace sound clinical decision-making.

References

Argenta LC, Morykwas MJ (1997) Vacuum-assisted closure: a new method for treatment: clinical experience. *Ann Plastic Surg* **38**(6): 563–76

Bale S (1997) A guide to wound debridement. *J Wound Care* **6**: 179–82

Banwell PE (1999) Topical negative pressure therapy in wound care. *J Wound Care* **8**(2): 79–84

Bishop SM, Walker M, Rogers AA, Chen WYJ (2003) Importance of moisture balance at the wound–dressing interface. *J Wound Care* **12**(4): 125–8

Bolton L, Hermans MHE (2004) How do we manage critically colonized wounds? *Rehabil Nurs* **29**(6): 187–94

Bowler PG (2002) Wound pathophysiology, infection and therapeutic options. *Ann Med* **34**(6): 419–27

Bowler P, Duerden B, Armstrong D (2001) Wound microbiology and associated approaches to wound management. *Clin Microbiol Rev* **14**(2): 244–69

Cameron J, Powell S (1992) Contact dermatitis: its importance in leg ulcer patients. *Wound Management* **2**(3): 12–13

Casadevall A, Pirofski L-A (2000) Host-pathogen interactions: basic concepts of microbial commensalism, colonization, infection and disease. *Infect Immun* **68**(12): 6511–18

Chen WY, Rogers AA, Lydon MJ (1992) Characterization of biologic properties of wound fluid collected during early stages of wound healing. *J Invest Dermatol* **99**(5): 559–64

Colebrook L, Lowbury EJ, Hurst L (1960) The growth and death of wound bacteria in serum, exudate and slough. *J Hyg* (Lond) **58**: 357–66

Cooper RA (2004) http://www.worldwidewounds.com/2004/february/Cooper/Topical-Antimicrobial-Agents.html

Cooper P, Russell F, Stringfellow S (2003) Modern wound management: an update of common products. *Nurs Residential Care* **5**(7): 322–34

Cutting KF (1999) The causes and prevention of maceration of the skin. *J Wound Care* **8**(4): 200–2

Cutting KF (2004) Wound exudate. In: White RJ, ed. *Trends in Wound Care, vol III*. Quay Books, MA Healthcare Ltd, London

Cutting K, Harding KG (1994) Criteria for identifying wound infection. *J Wound Care* **3**(4): 198–201

Cutting KF, White RJ (2005) Criteria for identifying wound infection: revisited. *Ostomy Wound Management* **5**(1): 28–34

Cutting KF, White RJ, Mahoney P, Harding KG (2005) *Identifying Criteria for Wound Infection*. Position document. EWMA, London

Cuzzell JZ (1988) The new red, yellow, black color code. *Am J Nurs* **88**(10): 1342–46

Davidson JM (1992) Wound repair. In: Gallin JI, Goldstein IM, Snyderman R, eds. *Inflammation: Basic Principles and Clinical Correlates*. 2nd edn. Raven Press, New York: 809–19

Davies P (2004) Current thinking on the management of necrotic and sloughy wounds. *Prof Nurse* **19**(10): 34–6

Dow G, Browne A, Sibbald RG (1999) Infection in chronic wounds: controversies in diagnosis and treatment. *Ostomy Wound Management* **45**(8): 23–7, 29–40

Dowsett C, Ayello E (2004) TIME principles of chronic wound bed preparation and treatment. *Br J Nurs* **13**(15): S16–23

Dowsett C, Edwards-Jones V, Davies S (2004) Infection control for wound bed preparation. *Br J Community Nurs Supplement* **9**(9): TIME Suppl 12–17

Edwards R, Harding KG (2004) Bacteria and wound healing. *Curr Opin Infect Dis* **17**(2): 91–6

Ennis W, Meneses P (2000) Wound healing at the local level: the stunned wound. *Ostomy Wound Management* **46**(1A Suppl): 39S–48S

European Pressure Ulcer Advisory Panel (1999) Guidelines on treatment of pressure ulcers. *EPUAP Review* **1**(2): 31–3

European Tissue Repair Society (2003) Statements on important aspects of wound healing. *ETRS Bulletin* **10**: 2–3

Field C, Kerstein M (1994) Overview of wound healing in a moist environment. *Am J Surg* **167**(Suppl 1a): S25–S30

Gilchrist B (1999) Wound infection. In: Miller M, Glover D, eds. *Wound Management: Theory and Practice*. NT Books, London

Gray D, White RJ, Cooper P (2003) The wound healing continuum. In: White RJ, ed. *The Silver Book*. Quay Books, MA Healthcare Ltd, London

Gray D, White RJ, Cooper P, Kingsley AR (2005). Understanding applied wound management. *Wounds UK* **1**(1): 62–8

Hampton S (2005) Caring for sloughy wounds. *J Community Nurs* **19**(4): 30–4

Heggers JP, Haydon S, Ko F *et al* (1992) *Pseudomonas aeruginosa* exotoxin A: its role in retardation of wound healing: the 1992 Lindberg Award. *J Burn Care Rehab* **13**(5): 512–18

Heinzelmann M, Scott M, Lam T (2002) Factors predisposing to bacterial invasion and infection. *Am J Surg* **183**: 179–90

Isenberg HD (1998) Pathogenicity and virulence: another view. *Clin Microbiol Rev* **1**(1): 40–53

Jones V (2004) Wound bed preparation and its implication for practice: an educationalist viewpoint. *Applied Wound Management Supplement 1*, Wounds UK, Aberdeen

Kingsley A (2001) A proactive approach to wound infection. *Nurs Stand* **11**(15): 50–8

Kingsley A (2003) The Wound Infection Continuum and its application to clinical practice. *Ostomy Wound Management* **49** Suppl 7A: 1–7

Kingsley A (2005) Practical use of modern honey dressings in chronic wounds. In: White R, Cooper R, Molan P, eds. *Honey: A modern wound management product.* Wounds UK, Aberdeen: 57–8

Kubo M, Van de Water L, Plantefaber LC *et al* (2001) Fibrinogen and fibrin are anti-adhesive for keratinocytes: a mechanism for fibrin eschar slough during wound repair. *J Invest Dermatol* **117**(6): 1369–81

Lamke LO, Nilsson GE, Reithner HL (1997) The evaporative water loss from burns and water permeability of grafts and artificial membranes used in the treatment of burns. *Burns* **3**: 159–65

Leaper DJ (1994) Prophylactic and therapeutic role of antibiotics in wound care. *Am J Surg* **167**(1A): 15S–20S

Moore K (2005) VAC therapy: interactions in the healing process. *Wounds UK* **1**(1): 86–93

O'Brien M (2002) Exploring methods of wound debridement. *Br J Community Nurs* **10**(12): 14

Parnham A (2002) Moist wound healing: does the theory apply to chronic wounds. *J Wound Care* **11**(4): 143–6

Rogers AA, Burnett S, Moore JC, Shakespeare PG, Chen WY (1995) Involvement of proteolytic enzymes — plasminogen activators — in the pathophysiology of pressure ulcers. *Wound Rep Regen* **3**(3): 273–3

Schein M, Wittmann DH, Wise L, Condon RE (1997) Abdominal contamination, infection and sepsis, a continuum. *Br J Surg* **84**(2): 269–72

Schultz GS, Sibbald RG, Falanga V *et al* (2003) Wound bed preparation: a systematic approach to wound management. *Wound Rep Regen* **11** (Suppl 1): S1–28

Sibbald RG, Williamson D, Orsted H, *et al* (2000) Preparing the wound — Debridement, bacterial balance, and moisture balance. *Ostomy Wound Management* **46**: 14–35

Stephens P, Wall IB, Wilson MJ *et al* (2003) Anaerobic cocci populating the deep tissues of chronic wounds impair cellular wound healing responses in vitro. *Br J Dermatol* **148**(3): 456–66

Tong A (1999) The identification and treatment of slough. *J Wound Care* **8**(7): 338–9

Thomas S (1997) Wound exudate — who needs it? In: Cherry G, Harding KG, eds. *Management of Wound Exudate*. Proceedings of Joint Meeting of EWMA and ETRS, Oxford 1997. Churchill Communications, London: 1–5

Thomas S, Andrews A, Jones M (1998) The use of larval therapy in wound management. *J Wound Care* **7**: 442–52

Vowden K, Vowden P (2004) The role of exudate in the healing process: understanding exudate management. In: White RJ, ed. *Trends in Wound Care, vol III*. Quay Books, MA Healthcare Ltd, London

Vowden K, Vowden P (2003) Understanding exudate management and the role of exudate in the healing process. *Br J Nurs* **12**(20; Suppl): S4–S14

Vowden K, Vowden P (2004) The role of exudate in the healing process: understanding exudate management. In: White RJ, ed. *Trends in Wound Care, vol III*. Quay Books, MA Healthcare Ltd, London: 3–22

Wall IB, Davies CE, Hill KE *et al* (2002) Potential role of anaerobic cocci in impaired human wound healing. *Wound Repair Regen* **10**(6): 346–53

Watret L (1997) Know how: management of wound exudate. *Nurs Times* **93**(30): 38–9

White RJ (2001) Managing exudate. Part 1. *Nurs Times* **97**(9): XI– XIII

White RJ (2003) The wound infection continuum. In: White RJ, ed. *The Silver Book*. Quay Books, MA Healthcare Ltd, London

White R, Cutting KF (2003) Interventions to avoid maceration of the skin and wound bed. *Br J Nurs* **12**(20): 1186–1201

Wilson JW, Schurr MJ, Le Blanc CL *et al* (2002) Mechanisms of bacterial pathogenicity. *Postgrad Med J* **78**: 216–24

Winter GD (1962) Formation of the scab and the rate of epithelialisation of superficial wounds in the skin of the young domestic pig. *Nature* **193**: 293–4

Witkowski JA, Parish LC (1982) Histopathology of the decubitus ulcer. *J Am Acad Dermatol* **6**(6): 1014–21

Self-assessment exercises

Identify a patient you have been treating with a complex or chronic wound.

Apply the Wound Healing Continuum to this patient, and identify where on the continuum the wound is positioned.

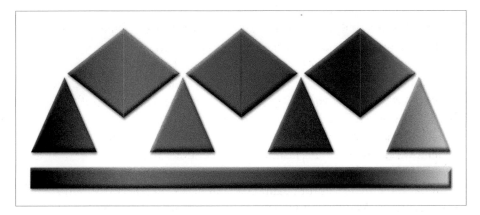

The Wound Healing Continuum

Where on the Wound Infection Continuum would this wound be situated?

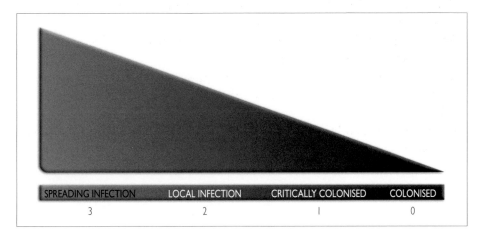

The Wound Infection Continuum

Can you say why this may be the case?

Using the Wound Exudate Continuum, score the wound moisture levels
and the viscosity of the exudate.

	VISCOSITY		
VOLUME	HIGH 5	MEDIUM 3	LOW 1
HIGH 5			
MEDIUM 3			
LOW 1			

The Wound Exudate Continuum

What was your treatment plan for the patient?

Would you change this treatment based on using the Applied Wound
Management assessment tool?

CHAPTER 5

APPLIED WOUND MANAGEMENT AS PART OF MEDICAL/NURSING MANAGEMENT

David Gray

Introduction

Applied Wound Management is just one element in the successful management of a patient with a wound. Today, patients with wounds tend to have chronic diseases such as cardiac failure, diabetes, renal disease, peripheral vascular disease (PVD) and cancer, to name but a few. These diseases can severely impact on the ability of the wound to heal along the lines of normal physiology (*Chapter 1*). Many of these diseases contribute to the factors which can delay healing (*Chapter 3*). The patient would be receiving less than optimal management if we were to treat the wound without acknowleding the impact of these factors. When assessing a patient with a wound and planning their care/management, it is vital that we do so as part of the mutlidisciplinary team, thereby ensuring that we utilise all the skills available within the team. Communication is a key element in this process, and members of the team, such as medical staff and other nursing staff who may not be reviewing the wound regularly, should be kept abreast of the wound's condition and any concurrent diseases.

In the two cases which follow, the seven key questions posed in *Chapter 4* (*pp. 73–75*) have been asked at first review of the patient. It may also be useful to refer to the tables in *Chapter 4* regarding products and their use in achieving various treatment objectives, to try and identify those you think would be most beneficial in each case.

Case 1: Elderly female

1.What kind of wound am I looking at?

This lady has presented with acute cellulitis of both lower limbs; the focus of this review is the right leg. The ulceration apparent in *Figure 5.1* is due to the spreading infection, and the yellow slough is a result of death of the superficial layers of the skin and the large volume of exudate being produced.

2. Why has this wound developed?

This wound has developed as a result of an infection in the leg, which has spread through the tissue resulting in the development of a systemic illness. The situation has been complicated by the presence of cardiac failure causing odema in both lower limbs.

3. What else is happening to this person?

This patient is morbidly obese, has cardiac failure, and also lives in challenging social circumstances. She has been admitted to an acute ward for the third time in twelve months for the treatment of lower limb cellulitis, and is currently systemically ill and receiving intravenous antibiotics.

4. What are the potential outcomes for the person with this wound?

Systemic infections can be life-threatening and it is vital that this patient receives urgent medical intervention with antibiotic therapy and management of her cardiac failure, to ensure that this illness does not develop into a life-threatening condition. With the correct systemic treatment and topical wound management, this patient has every possibility of achieving full healing. Ideally, her treatment after healing will involve compression hosiery to reduce the likelihood of recurrence.

5. What is the best management for this person?

The ideal management for this patient is a multidisciplinary approach, ensuring that the spreading infection is treated systemically while the wound is managed in such a way as to reduce the risk of re-infection. Topical antimicrobial products should be used to reduce the bacterial loading, together with absorptive products to prevent the wound exudate from lying on the wound surface and peri-wound areas. Finally, to reduce the risk of re-infection, a product which removes the slough which can act as a source of bacteria should be applied. The best management will also involve accurate medical management of the underlying cardiac failure. Once healing has been achieved, the vascular system in the limb should be assessed using either a Doppler ultrasound scan, or a duplex scan, to identify if the patient is suitable for compression hosiery. Compression hosiery can help to prevent a recurrence of the lower limb swelling by encouraging venous return, thereby reducing the risk of infection.

6. Do I have the skills to manage this person's wound?

Each practitioner should ask this question and be sure that they have the skills and knowledge needed to provide the best possible care for the patient. If not, seek advice or refer to a specialist.

7. How will I monitor the progress of this wound?

By utilising Applied Wound Management's clinical tools (Gray *et al*, 2005), the wound can be assessed in a systematic manner and accurately documented, facilitating ongoing assessment and evaluation. This includes ensuring that the dimensions of the wound are accurately measured and documented. It is also important that the patient's overall condition, relating to their nutrition, pain, mobility, etc are considered as part of their medical/nursing management.

Wound assessment			
	First review	Second review	Third review
Wound Healing Continuum	Yellow	Yellow/red	Pink
Wound Infection Continuum	Spreading	Localised	Colonised
Wound Exudate Continuum	High/medium	High/low	Low/low
Wound type	Leg ulcer	Leg ulcer	Leg ulcer
Treatment objectives	Debride Reduce bacterial loading Absorb moisture	Debride/ granulation Reduce bacterial loading Absorb moisture	Assess for compression hosiery Moisturise skin Prevent recurrence

Discussion

In this case, the patient has a life-threatening condition with her underlying cardiac failure. The spreading infection requires a systemic response but this can be enhanced by good wound management, which reduces the risks of re-infection while also promoting healing and lessening the pain. For the most beneficial outcome for the patient, both strategies need to be delivered together with good interdisciplinary communication. In *Figure 5.1a*, two legs are presented. The patient's right leg is the most severely affected, and the cellulitis can be seen spreading above the knee. In *Figure 5.1b* we can observe the slough which has been deposited on the surface of the wound, proving the ideal source of bacteria to re-infect the patient if left unattended. At the next review one week later, we can see in *Figures 5.2a* and *5.2b* that the slough has been removed and, while a small amount remains, the wound shows signs of improvement. In the final image (*Figure 5.3*), the right leg has now completely healed and has been managed with compression hosiery which is reducing the level of oedema in the limb and the risk of recurrence.

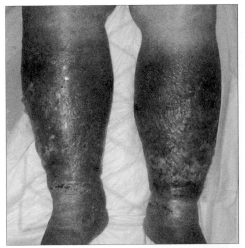

Figure 5.1a: Both legs show signs of cellulitis with the infection advancing above the knee on the right leg. The underlying cardiac failure has also contributed to the swelling on the legs

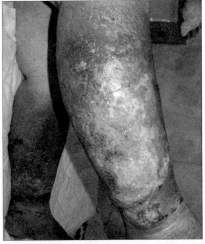

Figure 5.1b: The right leg has developed slough as a result of the blistering associated with the infection

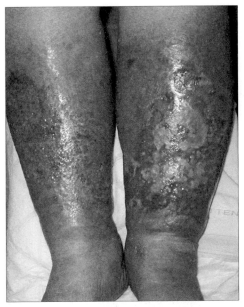

Figure 5.2a: At the second review the infection has reduced and is localised to the lower leg and some of the underlying swelling has been reduced

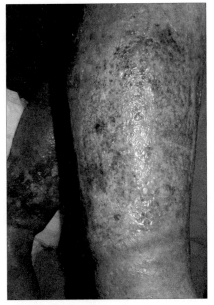

Figure 5.2b: The outer aspect of the right leg has now had most of the slough removed and the wound is developing new granulation tissue

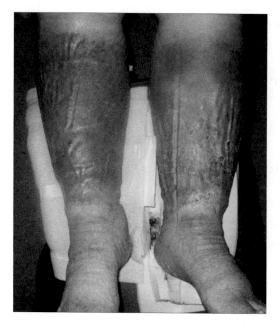

Figure 5.3: The right leg has now healed and is about to be fitted with compression hosiery in an effort to prevent lower limb swelling and reduce the risk of a recurrence of the cellulitis

Case 2: Elderly female

1.What kind of wound am I looking at?

This wound is a pressure ulcer which has developed on the left heel of an elderly lady who has suffered a stroke and is rehabilitating in hospital.

2. Why has this wound developed?

This wound has developed as a result of unrelieved pressure applied to the heel. This occurred during the acute phase of the patient's illness when she was unable to move her limbs sufficiently to maintain adequate circulation to the tissue.

3. What else is happening to this person?

She currently has reduced mobility, lower limb oedema and type 2 diabetes. As potential barriers to healing, all of these factors may reduce her ability to heal.

4. What are the potential outcomes for the person with this wound?

This wound can heal if the issues identified as barriers to healing are managed successfully, and the topical wound management is effective. However, failure to reduce localised oedema or remove devitalised tissue, could see the wound develop an infection which would delay healing.

5. What is the best management for this person?

Removing or reducing the barriers to healing will require a multi-disciplinary approach; in turn, this requires effective communication between nursing and medical teams concerning the localised oedema and diabetic management. The individual's seating position will need addressing to prevent any further pressure damage, with the provision of a mattress and some form of heel protection, such as a Repose™ Heel Boot (Frontier Therapeutics).

Management of the wound will require the removal of the devitalised tissue and the promotion of granulation tissue. This can be assessed using the Wound Healing Continuum (*Chapter 4, p. 76*). The levels of bacteria and moisture in the wound can be assessed using the Wound Infection and Wound Exudate Continuums respectively.

In summary, the ideal management will involve a multidisciplinary approach towards her immobility and diabetes, and accurate assessment and appropriate management of her wound.

6. Do I have the skills to manage this person's wound?

Each practitioner should ask this question and be sure that they have the skills and knowledge needed to provide the best possible care for the patient. If not, seek advice or refer to a specialist.

7. How will I monitor the progress of this wound?

By utilising Applied Wound Management's clinical tools (Gray *et al*, 2005), the wound can be assessed in a systematic manner and accurately documented, facilitating ongoing assessment and evaluation. This includes ensuring that the dimensions of the wound are accurately measured and documented. It is also important that the patient's overall condition, relating to her nutrition, pain, mobility, etc are considered as part of their medical/nursing management.

Wound assessment				
	First review	Second review	Third review	Fourth review
Wound Healing Continuum	Black/yellow	Yellow/red	Red	Red/pink
Wound Infection Continuum	Colonised	Colonised	Colonised	Colonised
Wound Exudate Continuum	Moderate/low	Low/low	Low/low	Low/low
Wound type	Pressure ulcer	Pressure ulcer	Pressure ulcer	Pressure ulcer
Treatment objectives	Debride/ granulation	Debride/ granulation	Granulation/ epithelialisation	Granulation/ epithelialisation
Treatment options	Refer to Chapter 4, Table 4.2, p. 93	Refer to Chapter 4, Table 4.2, p. 93	Refer to Chapter 4, Table 4.2, p. 93	Refer to Chapter 4, Table 4.2, p. 93

Discussion

From *Figure 5.4* it can be seen that at first review the patient has a large wound across the back of her heel. By using the Applied Wound Management system the requirement is to debride the black/yellow tissue from the wound, while promoting granulation. In *Figure 5.5* we can see that while slough remains in the wound bed, the black tissue has been removed and the patient has moved along the Wound Healing Continuum to yellow/red. In *Figure 5.6*, this process has continued and on the left of the wound, healing is being achieved faster than on the right. Finally, in *Figure 5.7*, one half of the wound has completely healed and the other half is granulating and closing.

The healing observed is a result of the management of the underlying diabetes and localised odema, which is the result of a multidisciplinary response. Effective wound management has been employed and its benefit maximised by managing the underlying factors which may delay healing.

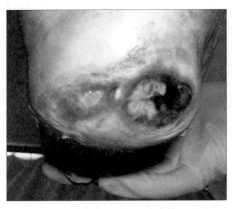

Figure 5.4: At the first review the wound covers most of the base of the heel and has necrotic/sloughy tissue across the majority of the wound bed, with granulating tissue at the margins

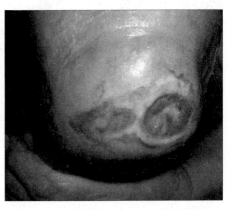

Figure 5.5: At the second review the wound has progressed along the Wound Healing Continuum and, in the centre of the wound, a bridge of epithelium has developed, dividing the wound into two separate wounds

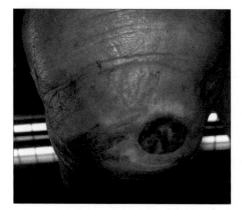

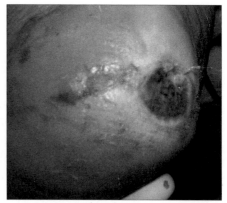

Figure 5.6: At the third review it can be seen that, having divided into two wounds, the wound on the left-hand side (of the patient) has now almost healed, and the wound on the right-hand side is filled almost entirely with granulating tissue

Figure 5.7: In this final assessment, the wound on the left-hand side has healed, and the wound on the right-hand side is granulating well with evidence of new epithelium at the margins and contraction of the granulating tissue

Reference

Gray D, McGuffog J, Cooper P, White R, Kingsley A (2005) Applied Wound Management: clinical tools to facilitate implementation. *Wounds UK* **1**(2) (Applied Wound Management supplement: Part 2): 25–30

INDEX